WHAT OTHERS SAY ABOUT
THE FOOD BIBLE

"I recommend The Food Bible *for anyone seeking better health through the foods they eat. Foods without preservatives and texturizers are much more healthy for the human body. I firmly believe in the principle that basic medicine should come from the farm and not the pharmacy."*

Howard E. Hagglund, M.D.

ɔↄ

"The Food Bible *eliminates questions for the health-conscious person . . . Taking* The Food Bible *to the grocery store makes shopping easier and provides an excellent resource for anyone selecting foods directly from the grocery shelves that are nutritious and free of additives and preservatives.* The Food Bible, *together with Jayne Benkendorf's advice in the newsletter,* Product Research Update, *not only includes nutritional information on specific foods, but also helps in daily diet planning."*

Nelda Fister, M.S., R.N.
Asst. Professor of Nursing
Central State University

"My son has a number of allergies, and I have found Jayne Benkendorf's book, The Food Bible, *to be extremely helpful in weeding out so many of the foods with additives. Jayne is one of the most thorough individuals I've ever met."*

Carole Howard
Belmont, California

❧

"Since I have an elevated cholesterol count, I have to be very careful of the foods I eat. I constantly use The Food Bible *to help me make wise choices."*

Betty Roberts

❧

"The simple-to-read, simple-to-use material in The Food Bible *has challenged our whole family toward the goal of eating to live instead of living to eat!"*

Kay Hill

❧

"By choice we are on a low-fat, low-sugar and low-salt diet. The Food Bible *has been a tremendous help because we have not had to do the research ourselves. We use it like we do any other encyclopedia — as a guide. The changes we have made would have been much more difficult without* The Food Bible."

Rita Crockett and Edwin Miller

THE FOOD BIBLE

by

JAYNE BENKENDORF

Library of Congress Cataloging-in-Publication Data

Benkendorf, Jayne, 1940-
    The food bible / Jayne Benkendorf
        p.   cm.
    Includes index.
    ISBN: 0-935834-77-X : $16.95
    1. Food--Composition--Popular works.   2. Nutrition--Popular works.
    I. Title.
    TX533.B38   1991
    641.1--dc20   91-8307
                                                                      CIP

THE FOOD BIBLE
By Jayne Benkendorf
Copyright 1991 by Jayne Benkendorf
Produced by Ratzlaff & Associates
Cover by Therese Cabell
Published by Rainbow Books, Inc.
P. O. Box 1069
Moore Haven, Florida 33471

Printed in the United States of America
Price: $16.95

WARNING/DISCLAIMER:

TABLE OF CONTENTS

FOREWORD
TO
THE FOOD BIBLE

The last ten (10) years have been witness to an explosion of information addressing the relationship between diet and health. These data run the gamut from speculation to clearly defined guidelines that have evolved from scientific research. Jayne Benkendorf has assembled a concise handbook that should prove to be very useful to any individual interested in taking a more active role in maintaining good health. *The Food Bible* offers a practical guide that simplifies and explains many of the currently held theories relating diet to disease.

C. H. Jameson, III, M.D.
Practicing Medical Oncologist
Tennessee

INTRODUCTION
TO
THE FOOD BIBLE

The Food Bible is a quick and easy reference guide for selecting healthful grocery products. Through a very unique rating system, I am able to rate grocery products for *Fat, Salt, Sugar, Cholesterol, Additives, Preservatives* and if *Highly Processed.* With *The Food Bible* we can quickly check our favorite foods to see how they rate. So often I have found two different brands of a food sitting side by side on a grocery shelf — one has ingredients that are very healthful and the other is what I call "a health hazard." *The Food Bible* tells us which one is the best choice. With *The Food Bible*, we can see that certain manufacturers are more concerned than others about the healthfulness of their products. One takes pride in what they offer while the other apparently is interested in only one thing   making money. Through advertising, two manufacturers can make their products look like they have health written all over them. In reality, one may be very good and the other may be loaded with questionable ingredients. *The Food Bible* will identify which is best.

WHO USES *THE FOOD BIBLE?*

I have found, through field testing, that during the course of a year, nearly every family will look for better products to feed themselves and their family. With some food shoppers, it is almost a daily task, while others may search only a few times a year. Different things motivate different people toward a better quality of life through better nutrition. Weight control, constantly feeling tired and run down, chronic headaches, upset stomach, hyperactivity in children, coping with stress, and allergies are among conditions which motivate us to evaluate the quality of the food we are eating. For others, it may be fear. The fear of a high cholesterol count or a close friend or relative suffering from a heart attack; the fear of cancer, Alzheimer's Disease and other degenerative diseases; the fear that something is wrong because, "I'm constantly not feeling up to par." And yes, even the fear of premature aging. Now, with *The Food Bible*, we have a choice — a quick and easy reference guide for upgrading the quality of food we are eating. Even the American Heart Association and the American Cancer Society are now saying that what we eat may be our biggest health problem in the United States.

QUICK AND EASY TO USE

For many years I have been an advocate of nutritious, quick and easy cooking. I can remember so well the questions that I kept hearing over and over at the end of my cooking classes: *"I don't have time to read and analyze the ingredients in every food I buy. Isn't there some way you could do this for me?"* I guess when I heard the same statement so many times and for so long, I began to realize that there was a need.

That was over four years ago. During the past two years, when I initiated the field testing of *The Food Bible* concepts, those same demands kept reappearing. "I don't have a lot of time. I want something that will tell me which foods are the best, and it has to be quick and easy to use." These demands have been met. This is why a very unique rating system was designed and a rating code employed along with a simple layout that requires very little time to use.

RATING FOODS

I have found that food products basically fall into three categories:

Category I — These are foods which contain ingredients that we should avoid as much as possible. Foods containing any of these ingredients (see Chapter 1) are deemed not good enough to even get into *The Food Bible.*

Category II — These are foods which contain ingredients that we should limit. These products are listed in *The Food Bible* and are rated and coded for quick identification. These are *the high fat, high sodium and highly refined sugar foods; the highly processed foods; and the foods with significant cholesterol.* See Chapter 2 for details and why these foods should be limited.

Category III — These are foods which do not appear to have any use-limitations and are given a star (★) rating in *The Food Bible.*

POOL OF KNOWLEDGE

During the late 1960s, a financial advisory firm in Atlanta was conceived with a philosophy that made a lasting impression on me. Their basic philosophy is that no one person can possibly obtain enough schooling and experience to be considered "the authority" on a subject as diverse as finance. But rather, highly trained specialists in very defined areas of finance can pool their knowledge, creating a "real" authority in the field of finance.

I have used this "pool of knowledge" concept with regard to analyzing and rating food ingredients. My first concern when analyzing ingredients is to get the facts. I have relied upon specifically trained individuals and research institutions in the fields of medicine, nutrition, pharmacology, chemicals, food additives and preservatives and those with a special interest in food processing and distribution. With the background of trained specialists, the financial and research support from Product Research Service and my personal effort to the study of analyzing food ingredients, there is no doubt in my mind that *The Food Bible* is *"THE AUTHORITY."* Just like the financial institution in Atlanta, *The Food Bible* is our "real" authority in rating grocery products accurately and without bias.

I mentioned a special interest in food processing and distribution. Regardless of how much brain power we have at our disposal, "hands-on" experience is still necessary. This is why I have personally become very involved with the trip our food takes from the farm to the grocery store. Books don't teach what I have learned; and believe me, I can tell some hair-raising stories. It is through this trip (from the farm to the grocery shelf) that the quality of the food we're eating is determined.

I certainly learned firsthand what is meant by the expression, "They've taken all the food out of this food." I was told very candidly by an employee of a large manufacturing company how they develop a new food product. First, they make certain that it contains plenty of the two tastes Americans love — fat and salt. Then they add just enough "real" food to make it look and sound healthful. Next they give it a catchy name so it will sell. At the other end of the scale, I saw a company wanting to provide even better quality products than government regulations allow. Fortunately, I see this latter mentality growing. We, the consumer, have the choice, and *The Food Bible* gives us the tool for making these better choices.

AS WE DEMAND GOOD FOODS, SO WILL THE NUMBER OF GOOD FOODS INCREASE ON OUR GROCERY SHELVES.

CHAPTER 1
FOODS WE
SHOULD AVOID

Most health professionals spend full time treating and administering medicine for diseases such as: heart disease, cancer, arthritis, diabetes, hypertension, headaches, etc. Yet, at the same time, a new generation of health professionals is emerging with a focus on *cause*. Why are we, as a society, being plagued with a myriad of degenerative diseases, and what can be done to reverse this trend? Evidence is mounting that at the rate we're going today, in 20 years, 50% of the people in the United States can expect to have cancer in their lifetime. What is causing this trend? More and more we are finding that the foods we are eating are at the root of the problem. Evidence is pouring in which shows that **what we eat does make a difference**.

Let's look at some real shocking statistics. It is estimated that during the past 50 years:

Pastry consumption has increased	70%
Soft drink consumption has increased	80%
Potato chip consumption has increased	85%
Fat consumption has increased	100%
Salt consumption has increased	100%
Sugar consumption has increased	100%
Vegetable consumption has decreased	40%
Fruit consumption has decreased	45%
Whole grain consumption has decreased	150%

All this has happened during a time when cancer has increased some 150%. As startling as these figures may seem, the one that I feel is most noteworthy is this:

Since World War II, we have increased our consumption of chemically altered foods from 10% to 80% of our total diet.

Never in the history of mankind has the human body been exposed to such an array of unnatural and synthetic foods, and virtually all of this has been dumped on us in the past 45 years. It is little wonder why some health professionals are now realizing that, "Hey, maybe we have gotten off the track," and they are going back to basics and looking at what nature intended our bodies to receive.

Synthetic and chemically prepared additives and preservatives in our foods are at an all time high. Does this mean that all are bad? No, but knowing which ones are safe can, at best, be tricky. Testing is required before new additives and preservatives can be used, but a two- or three-year test on mice does not always tell us what effects 20 years of consuming an additive will have on humans. So even though chemicals are approved for use in our foods, testing continues; and if sufficient damaging evidence is forthcoming, its use will be discontinued.

At least that's the way it's supposed to work. For example, in 1977, saccharin, an artificial sweetener, was deemed unsafe for human consumption by scientists in Canada, Great Britain and the United States. Canada and Great Britain immediately curtailed its use; but in the United States, because of a tremendous public outcry, the FDA was swayed, and they allowed saccharin use to continue, but with a warning that it may be harmful.

This type of mentality has prevailed, and over the past ten to fifteen years there are, in my opinion, a number of additives and preservatives that are very dangerous if consumed over a period of time. The Delaney Clause, which was passed in 1958, stated that "no additive shall be deemed to be safe if it is found to induce cancer when ingested by man or animal, or if it is found, after test., which are appropriate for the evaluation of the safety of food ϝ ιditives, to induce cancer in man or animal." Since the advent of the saccharin incident in 1977, the FDA has been unable to ɛnforce the Delaney Clause, and a number of additives and preservatives are currently being used, without restrictions, that would otherwise cause them to be banned under the terms of the Delaney Clause. These are additives and preservatives that have been proven or are suspected to cause health problems, but for reasons stated, are still in our foods.

Based on my research, I have identified in this chapter which of these additives and preservatives are the most dangerous and should be avoided. These are additives and preservatives which are suspected of causing cancer, brain damage, hyperactivity, allergies, headaches, hypertension and a number of other degenerative diseases.

Following is an alphabetical listing of each additive and preservative and a short explanation about why I deem each to be potentially unsafe. Because of these potential dangers involved, no foods thought to contain any of these additives and preservatives will knowingly be included in *The Food Bible*.

ALGINATES
(ammonium, calcium, potassium and sodium; propylene glycol alginate; algin derivatives)

Alginates are used to stabilize and promote a creamy texture in foods. The sodium form of alginate seems to be the most suspect, and the FDA is performing tests for childbirth and reproductive problems.

Alginates are used in products such as ice cream, ices, salad dressings, cheese spreads, frozen dinners, ramen soups and others.

ALUMINUM

Aluminum destroys brain cells, and aluminum deposits have been found in the brains of Alzheimer's victims. Dr. Lowell L. Henderson of the Mayo Clinic does admit that extra aluminum is present in the brains of many Alzheimer's victims, but he believes that the extra aluminum is caused by the Alzheimer's disease itself. Other health professionals believe that aluminum may be part of the cause of Alzheimer's.

I want to share these two items with you: On the island of Guam, the aluminum deposits in the soil are unusually high, and there is a high incidence of Alzheimer's disease. Also, a recent report from the British government offers the strongest tie yet of aluminum to Alzheimer's disease. In areas of England and Wales where there are high levels of aluminum in drinking water, there is a marked increase in Alzheimer's disease.

We are exposed to aluminum in a number of ways. In addition to being added to many foods, we also see it in beer and soda pop cans and in the packaging of many products.

Aluminum has its benefits with packaging in that it helps retain freshness. I have no problem with packaging unless the product is of an acid nature such as citrus juices, etc. The acid eats into and absorbs some of the aluminum. In my opinion, beer and pop cans are very suspect as both are acidic and leach aluminum from the can. Glass bottles are always a better choice.

Another area where aluminum appears to be showing up is in some processed cheeses. Manufacturers are not required to list the ingredients of cheeses, so it is difficult to detect. I had some random selections of cheese tested and found that the American processed varieties had the highest concentrations of aluminum. I understand that it is added for melting purposes.

I do not believe that there is enough aluminum in any one source to be that concerned about — unless we overconsume that one source, such as drinking a lot of soda pop or beer from aluminum cans. However, aluminum is beginning to show up in more and more of our products, and this really does concern me.

Aluminum tends to accumulate in our bodies over the years — which is an explanation for its association with Alzheimer's disease. Therefore, it is my opinion, that we should avoid, as much as possible, products that contain aluminum. *The Food Bible* does not include any known products where the labeling reveals that aluminum has been added. However, I do want to caution you. Even though cheeses are included in *The Food Bible*, it is my opinion that our processed cheeses, such as American singles, Velveeta, the Lite Naturals, cheese sauces and spreads as well as most grated parmesans, are very suspect at containing higher than normal levels of aluminum. For this reason, you may choose to limit their use.

ARTIFICIAL COLORS

There are many colors approved for use in our foods with nearly half of them artificial. Many artificial colors are made of coal-tar based (azo) dyes. Artificial colors are used because many natural colors turn pale with time. For example, butter turns a pale yellow and some fruits in ice creams turn dark. Manufacturers soon learned that these artificial colors made customers think products were better, and they learned that they could take an inferior product, color it and it would look wholesome and fresh. They also realize that children are attracted to these bright colors and will encourage their parents to buy only the bright ones. So the artificial color industry became an instant success — and as a bonus, artificial colors are cheaper than their natural counterparts.

Over the years though, many artificial colors have been banned by the FDA and some four to seven colors now in use are suspect. Concerns include malignancy, toxicity, allergic reactions, hyperactivity in children, etc. Some colors such as red #40, red #3, citrus red #2, yellow #5, yellow #6, and blue #2 are most suspect. But the history of all artificial colors is not that good, so I feel it is in our best interest to avoid all foods with artificial coloring. They have absolutely no purpose in food except to make them appear better than they are. I am particularly concerned with so many children's products containing these artificial colors. Foods notorious for artificial colors include: drink mixes, puddings, cereals, candy, gelatin desserts, ice cream, etc.

ARTIFICIAL FLAVORS

There are around 1,500 artificial flavors used in our food. When natural flavors are removed through processing, artificial ones are used to replace them. This is the largest category of additives in our foods. (Some names include: benzaldehyde and methyl salicylates.) None is thought to be life threatening; however, artificial flavors such as benzyl alcohol, butyl acetate and benzaldehyde have been associated with depression and reduced sexual urges. Some have also been associated with reproductive problems, and a link between hyperactivity in children and artificial flavors has been proven. We do not need to be inflicting these potential problems on our bodies. There are too many natural flavorings to choose from such as: lemon, orange, grape, and all the spices, etc.

BENZOIC ACID
(sodium benzoate)

Benzoic acid and its salt, sodium benzoate, can affect the nervous system, can cause allergic reactions, asthma attacks, stomach irritations and hyperactivity in children. They are used as preservatives and also as antifungal agents. Conflicting reports regarding their safety exist, so any products found to include benzoic acid and sodium benzoate are not included in *The Food Bible*.

Foods containing benzoic acid and sodium benzoate include margarines, baked goods, juices, ices, ice creams, frozen dinners and others.

BHA & BHT
(butylated hydroxyanisole and
butylated hydroxytoluene)

BHA and BHT both are preservatives and antioxidants and are used to keep foods from changing color and to keep fats from becoming rancid. Both can cause allergic reactions, can affect the nervous system, and precipitate behavioral problems in children. Research has shown that mice, when fed a ration of one half of one percent of either BHA or BHT, gave birth to offspring with abnormal behavior patterns. A real concern with BHA and BHT is how they affect liver and kidney functions. Experiments at Michigan State University suggest that BHT is more toxic to the kidneys than BHA. In fact, BHT is completely banned in all foods in England. Both BHA and BHT are suspect in causing increased susceptibility to cancer-causing agents. The Select Committee of the American Society for Experimental Biology has advised the FDA to perform further studies regarding the affects BHT has when used in conjunction with hormones and oral contraceptives. Evidence suggests that BHT, at levels now permitted in foods, may convert hormones and oral contraceptives into carcinogenic agents. In my opinion, these are two potentially very dangerous preservatives, especially BHT — and hopefully both will be banned soon.

Foods most likely to contain either BHA or BHT include: cereals, baked goods, drink mixes, instant potato flakes, boxed dinners, chewing gum and others.

BROMATE
(calcium bromate and potassium bromate)

Calcium bromate and potassium bromate are dough conditioners and can affect the function of the kidneys as well as the nervous system. An outbreak of food poisoning in New Zealand was the result of sugar being contaminated with potassium bromate. Bromates appear to be very toxic if the dosage becomes too high; in fact, the lethal dosage is not even known. Although very small amounts appear to be fairly safe, to my knowledge, no research has been performed concerning the possible buildup of bromate poison in our bodies. Common foods that contain bromates include bread, baked goods, packaged bread crumbs, refrigerated biscuits and others.

COTTONSEED OIL

Some studies indicate that cottonseed oil may contribute to infertility in males. However, my concern here is with cotton as a crop. Since cotton is not a food crop, chemicals banned for use on food crops do not apply to cotton. The problem with cotton seems to be at harvest time. It is much easier for farmers to pick their cotton if the plants have been defoliated. So how do you get green leaves to dry up and fall off? You apply a chemical. A restricted chemical, paraquat, (requiring a special license to use), has been and still is being used for defoliation. This chemical can be extremely dangerous if it is breathed or if it comes in contact with the skin. Some licensed applicators will not use it because they fear for their own safety.

But guess what is being used as a substitute? Arsenic! This may be even worse than paraquat as far as cottonseed oil is concerned. In fact, there was a big stink among the ranks regarding residues of this chemical that may still be in cotton clothes. I feel that this issue will be resolved, but farmers will simply find some other chemical to get their defoliating done.

The cottonseed oil comes from the cotton seed which is inside the little balls of cotton on the top of each sprayed plant. Most cotton seed is processed into cattle feed, except for the small amount that is used for cottonseed oil. I believe that the risk of possible dangerous chemical residues is too great to recommend any foods where cottonseed oil is used.

Products that contain cottonseed oil include: crackers, soups, salad dressings, cookies, baking mixes, potato chips, etc.

DISODIUM GUANYLATE AND DISODIUM INOSINATE

Both are flavor enhancers and are generally used in combination. They can increase uric acid concentrations and can precipitate gout. Most products that include disodium guanylate and disodium inosinate have already been excluded from *The Food Bible* because of other additives and preservatives. Disodium guanylate and disodium inosinate are found in products such as salad dressings, boxed and frozen dinners, crackers, ramen soups and others.

EDTA
(ethylenediamine tetra-acetic acid)

EDTA is used as a metal deactivator. It attracts metallic contaminants brought about by food processing. EDTA binds with metal particles and removes them from the body. In the process, it also removes other metals which are vital to our health such as iron, zinc, etc. Because of this mineral loss, it is especially important for pregnant and nursing women to avoid foods with EDTA. The FDA is currently conducting further studies for toxicity and kidney damage.

Foods containing EDTA include: margarine, salad dressings, canned legumes, boxed dinners, frozen dinners and others.

MSG
(monosodium glutamate)

MSG is a very taste-appealing, sodium-based flavor enhancer. MSG is traditionally associated with Chinese foods and Chinese restaurants. The term "Chinese Restaurant Syndrome" came about because many people, after eating Chinese foods, suffered from chest pain, headaches, a burning sensation in the neck area, diarrhea, stomach cramping, joint pain similar to arthritis, weakness, slurred speech and a number of other discomforts. In addition to Chinese foods, we are seeing more and more MSG use in other foods. Manufacturers have learned that MSG will greatly increase the flavors of certain highly processed foods, especially those where salt flavoring is compatible.

MSG really is quite amazing in what it can do for the taste of food, but serious concerns about its safety are questioned. Baby food processors have already removed MSG from their products because of public concern, and the FDA has been instructed to perform further studies. The most serious concerns relate to its possible cancer-causing effects, reproduction and fertility effects, and its possible brain-altering effects.

In addition to Chinese foods, the following type foods contain MSG: seasoned salt, soups, bouillon, frozen dinners, salad dressing mixes, boxed dinners and others.

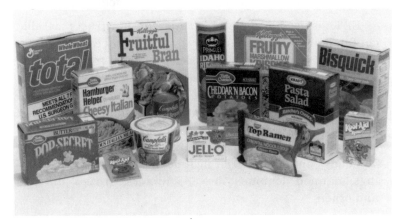

Foods containing additives and preservatives.

NITRATES AND NITRITES

Sodium nitrite is found more frequently in our food products than sodium nitrate, and it is used as a preservative primarily in cured meats. It gives a distinctive taste and pink color to bacon, bologna, salami, frankfurters, ham, potted meats, pepperoni, etc. Nitrites combine with stomach juices to form powerful cancer-causing agents called nitrosamines. Nitrites and nitrates are used in meats to kill botulism spores, a very deadly bacteria. However, scientists tell us that other processing methods can be used just as effectively as nitrites, but they would not impart the taste and color that consumers are used to. The meat would be a gray color instead of pink, and the taste wouldn't be the same. (I know that I'd rather have a gray piece of ham than cancer!) If we were accustomed to eating gray ham and someone said we had to start eating pink ham, you know we'd throw a fuss.

A note from the National Research Council:

"Several chemical and physical treatments appear to be comparable in inhibiting outgrowth of 'clostridium botulinum' spores in types of meat products but none confers the color and flavor that consumers have come to expect in nitrite-cured meats."

A quote from Michael F. Jacobson, director of Center for Science in the Public Interest, regarding nitrite:

"It is one of the most toxic chemicals in our food supply. Dozens of persons have died from nitrite poisoning and countless others have been incapacitated."

In 1978, the FDA and the U.S.D.A. announced that a study at M.I.T. (Massachusetts Institute of Technology) clearly demonstrated that nitrites cause cancer. I feel that eventually nitrates and nitrites will be completely banned.

NUTRASWEET
(aspartame)

NutraSweet, also known as Equal, is a sugar substitute which has the same number of calories as sugar but is 200 times sweeter. Aspartame was approved for use in dry food and as a table-top sweetener in 1981, and in 1983 its use was approved for soft drinks. As the result of research, two scientists in 1985 requested that labeling include the amount of aspartame in products. Research showed that children could suffer brain damage from a high intake of aspartame. Many obstetricians advise their patients not to consume products containing aspartame during pregnancy or when breast feeding because of the danger of brain damage to the fetus or infant. All products that contain aspartame must carry a warning to people with phenylketonuria (PKU) — a genetic disorder. Other problems that have been associated with aspartame include: headaches, dizziness, behavioral changes, mood swings, seizures, and urinary tract infections. Products that contain aspartame include: gelatin desserts, soft drinks, beverage mixes, hot cocoa mixes, desserts, yogurt and others.

POLYSORBATES
(sorbitol derivatives)

Polysorbates are emulsifiers and stabilizers. These have been associated with dioxane, a known carcinogen. They are undergoing further investigation. I choose not to include foods in *The Food Bible* that contain polysorbates because of unknowns; however, most foods that contain polysorbates have already been excluded because of other additives and preservatives.

Polysorbates are found most often in foods such as ice cream, non-dairy whipped toppings, non-dairy coffee whiteners, salad dressings, cakes, cake mixes and others.

POTASSIUM SORBATE

Potassium sorbate is a preservative and is used primarily as a yeast and mold inhibitor. It can affect the nervous system and can cause skin irritations. This is a preservative that does not appear to be that suspect; however, most food products that include potassium sorbate have already been excluded from *The Food Bible* because of other additives and preservatives.

Potassium sorbate is found primarily in baked goods, cheese spreads, margarines and desserts.

PROPIONIC ACID
(calcium propionate and sodium propionate)
Propionic acid and its compounds are preservatives used mainly to prevent mold. They do not appear to be life threatening; however, they may precipitate migraine headaches in those prone to get headaches, and they may affect the nervous system. Most food products that include propionic acid and its compounds have already been excluded from *The Food Bible* because they contain one or more of the higher risk additives and preservatives.

Foods which normally contain propionic acid include doughnuts, snack cakes, stuffing mixes, packaged bread crumbs and others.

PROPYL GALLATE
Propyl gallate is an antioxidant and is used primarily to keep fats from becoming rancid. So this means that we will find it most frequently in foods that contain fats. It is also used in many cosmetics — creams, lotions, lip balms, etc. — and can cause skin irritations.

In food products, we will find it used many times along with BHA and BHT because of the synergistic effects these three antioxidants have. Obviously, this compounds the problems that can occur.

Studies indicate that propyl gallate can cause allergic reactions and can precipitate asthmatic reactions. This means that people with allergies or asthma are at an increased risk when they eat foods with propyl gallate. Studies have also shown that propyl gallate can irritate the stomach, particularly in people who are sensitive to aspirin. Also, a very in-depth, long-term study indicates that propyl gallate may be cancer causing.

Common products that contain propyl gallate include boxed dinners and side dishes, granola bars, gravy mixes, turkey breakfast sausage and others.

PROPYLENE GLYCOL

Propylene glycol is an humectant, and as such its purpose is to hold moisture in products. Large doses in animals affect the nervous system and can cause kidney damage. It is also found in many cosmetic products and can irritate the skin. This additive does not appear to be that suspect; however, most food products that include propylene glycol have already been excluded from *The Food Bible* because they contain one or more other high risk additives or preservatives.

Propylene glycol can be found in shredded coconut, ice cream, icings, baked goods and others.

SACCHARIN

Saccharin is an artificial sweetener and has been found to cause malignant bladder tumors in laboratory animals. As a result, on March 9, 1977, the FDA announced that the use of saccharin in foods and beverages would be banned. This decision was based on a Canadian study which showed that seven out of 38 animals developed tumors, three of them malignant. In 1977, the American public was using so much of this artificial sweetener that they convinced the FDA not to ban saccharin. Saccharin continues to be in the market place, but products have warning labels saying that it may be hazardous to our health. The Committee of the Institute of Medicine and National Research Council, on November 6, 1978, reported that it had reached the conclusion that saccharin is a potential carcinogen *in humans*.

Saccharin is generally found in products advertising "low calories", "lite", etc., such as: desserts, soda pop, and it is used as a table-top sweetener.

SILICON DIOXIDE

Silicon dioxide is used as an anticaking agent and as a defoamer in beer. As a food additive, its use is restricted because the long-term effects of ingesting silicon dioxide have not been determined. Prolonged inhalation can cause lung damage.

Silicon dioxide can be found in such products as grated cheese, salt and salt substitutes and others.

SMOKED FOODS AND SMOKE FLAVORING

Smoke adds a distinctive flavor to foods, but this process of cooking can give us a very potent carcinogen similar to the tar in cigarette smoke. Fat that drips onto a fire or hot coals produces these carcinogens. If your lifestyle is one that finds you doing a lot of grilling or barbecuing, you may want to re-evaluate these practices. Repeated exposure obviously is where risk becomes greater. Some experts feel that if we grill over flames or coals, we can reduce our risk somewhat if we keep the temperature low and the food as far away from the heat source as possible.

Common foods which are smoked or include smoke flavoring are bacon, ham, turkey, chicken, cheese, fish, barbecue sauce and liquid smoke flavoring.

SULFITES
(sulfur dioxide, potassium bisulfite, sodium bisulfite, sodium sulfite, potassium metabisulfite, sodium metabisulfite)

Sulfites are preservatives and antioxidants that can be very dangerous for some people. They are permitted for use on all foods except fresh fruits and vegetables and any food high in vitamin B_1. They are not allowed on B_1 foods because sulfites destroy vitamin B_1. Although banned from fresh fruits and vegetables, some have been reported still in use, so it is suggested that outside leaves of lettuce, etc. should be destroyed. Also, ask if sulfites have been used.

Individuals who are particularly susceptible to sulfites are those affected with allergies and/or asthma. Symptoms may include severe headaches, facial and head flushing, abdominal pains and faintness. These symptoms, which can occur together or singly, generally occur rather quickly (15 to 30 minutes) after eating foods with sulfites. The FDA has confirmed 17 deaths due to sulfites. In a closed discussion in 1988, the FDA decided not to ban sulfites on certain foods sold in grocery stores and served in restaurants. Hopefully, this decision will be reviewed in the future, banning the complete use of sulfites.

In some cases, minute amounts of sulfites (those under ten parts per million) can be used on foods without labeling — which makes it impossible to completely police all foods. To the best of my knowledge, no foods are listed in *The Food Bible* which contain over ten parts per million of sulfites.

Sulfites, used to keep foods from discoloring, can be found in the following foods: dried fruits, cereals that contain dried fruit, children's fruit snacks, boxed dinners and others. They're also present in wine, wine coolers and beer.

TBHQ
(tertiary butylhydroquinone)

TBHQ is an antioxidant with a petroleum base that keeps foods from turning dark. It is used alone or in combination with BHA and/or BHT. The FDA has restricted its use to .02% of its oil and fat content because it can be quite toxic at higher levels causing nausea, vomiting and delirium. I choose not to include any known foods that contain this preservative; however, TBHQ by itself does not keep many foods out of *The Food Bible* since it is frequently used in conjunction with BHA and BHT — foods that I have already omitted.

The most common type foods which contain TBHQ include icings, stuffing mixes, refrigerated biscuits and microwave popcorn.

TROPICAL FATS AND LARD

The tropical fats include coconut oil, palm kernel oil and palm oil; lard is pure animal fat. These are the most highly saturated fats known, and the American Heart Association says that it is these fats that cause the greatest risk for heart disease. These forms of fat have generally been used in foods because they are very inexpensive and they do not become rancid quickly; therefore, we see them in many foods. Recently, however, public awareness of the dangers of these fats is causing some manufacturers to switch to other forms of fat that are less saturated.

Foods that I'm still seeing these tropical fats and lard used in include: cookies, crackers, snack cakes, baked goods, cereals, whipped toppings, baking mixes, frozen dinners, non-dairy creamers and others.

SUMMARY

Based on my research, these are the most dangerous of all additives and preservatives used in foods. For this reason, foods known to include any of these additives and preservatives are **not** included in *The Food Bible*.

Nearly every week I receive calls from clients telling me that since they are eating only foods listed in *The Food Bible* their headaches, digestive problems, diarrhea, etc. have stopped. If short-term use of additives and preservatives can cause these health problems, just imagine what long-term use may cause.

PROFESSIONAL REFERENCES AND
SUGGESTED READINGS

Alade, Soloman L., Ph.D., et al. "Polysorbate 80 and E-Ferol Toxicity." *Pediatrics*, 77 (April, 1986), pp. 593-597.

Allen, David H., M.B., Ph.D., John Delohery, M.B., and Gary Baker, M.B., B.Sc. *Journal of Allergy and Clinical Immunology*, 80 (2) (October, 1987), pp. 530-537.

Beasley, C.R.W., R.R.A.C.P., P. Rafferty, M.C.R.P., S. T. Holgate, M.D., F.R.C.P. "Bronchoconstrictor Properties of Preservatives in Ipratropium Bromide (Atrovent) Nebuliser Solution." *British Medical Journal*, 294 (6581) (May, 1987), pp. 1197-1198.

Berger, Stuart M. *Dr. Berger's Immune Power Diet.* New York: Signet New American Library, 1985.

Birchall, J.D., and J. S. Chappell. "The Chemistry of Aluminum and Silicon in Relation to Alzheimer's Disease." *Clinical Chemistry*, 34 (2) (February, 1988), pp. 265-267.

Brody, Jane. *Jane Brody's Nutrition Book.* New York: Bantam Books, 1987.

Dreher, Henry. *Your Defense Against Cancer.* New York: Harper & Row, 1988.

"Eating Clean²: Overcoming Food Hazards." *A Consumer's Guidebook.* Selected readings. Washington, D.C.: Center for Study of Responsive Law.

Feingold, Ben F., M.D. *Why Your Child Is Hyper-Active.* New York: Random House, 1974, 1975.

Fuchs, Nan Kathryn, Ph.D. *The Nutrition Detective.* Los Angeles: P. Tarcher, Inc., distributed by St. Martin's Press (New York), 1985.

Garland, Emily M., Takao Sakata, Maria J. Fisher, Tsuneo Masui, and Samuel M. Cohen. "Influences of Diet and Strain on the Proliferative Effect on the Rat Urinary Bladder Induced by Sodium Saccharin." *Cancer Research*, 49 (July 15, 1989), pp. 3789-3794.

Goldbeck, Nikki and David. *The Goldbeck's Guide to Good Food.* New York and Scarborough, Ontario: New American Library, 1987.

Gross, Peter A., M.D., Kendrick Lance, M.D., Robert Whitlock, M.D., and Ralph S. Blume, M.D. "Additive Allergy: Allergic Gastroenteritis Due to Yellow Dye #6." *Annals of Internal Medicine,* III (July, 1989), pp. 87-88.

Hadley, Allison. "Hazardous Cures." *Nursing Times,* 82 (39) (September 24-30, 1986), pp. 44-46.

Harrington, Geri. *Real Food Fake Food.* New York: Macmillan Publishing Company, Inc., 1987.

Hunter, Beatrice Trum. *The Mirage of Safety.* New York: Charles Scribner's Sons, 1975.

————. *The Sugar Trap.* Boston: Houghton Mifflin Company, 1982.

Jacobson, Michael F. *The Complete Eater's Digest and Nutrition Scoreboard.* Garden City, New York: Anchor Press/Doubleday, 1985.

————. *The Consumer's Factbook of Food Additives.* Garden City, New York: Doubleday and Company, Inc., 1972.

Johns, M.D., "Migraine Provoked by Aspartame." *New England Journal of Medicine,* 315 (August 14, 1986), p. 456.

Krishnan, S. S., D. R. McLachlan, B. Krishnan, S. S. Fenton, and J. E. Harrison. "Aluminum Toxicity to the Brain." *Science of the Total Environment,* 71 (1) (April, 1988), pp. 59-64.

Kulczycki, Anthony, Jr., M.D. "Aspartame-Induced Urticaria." *Annals of Internal Medicine,* 104 (February, 1986), pp. 207-208.

Lipton, Richard B., M.D., Lawrence C. Newman, M.D., Joel S. Cohen, M.D. and Seymour Soloman, M.D. "Aspartame as a Dietary Trigger of Headache." *Headache,* 29 (2) (February, 1989), pp. 90-92.

Lipton, Richard B., M.D., et al, Robert V. Steinmetzer, M.D., et al, Louis J. Elsas, II, M.D., and S. S. Schiffman, Ph.D., et al. "Aspartame and Headache." *New England Journal of Medicine,* 318 (May 5, 1988), pp. 1200-1202.

Livingston-Wheeler, Virginia. *The Conquest of Cancer.* New York, London, Toronto, Sydney: Franklin Watts, 1984.

Loewen, Gregory M., D.O., David Weiner, M.D., F.C.C.P., and
James McMahan, Ph.D. "Pneumoconiosis in an Elderly
Dentist." *Chest*, 93 (6) (June, 1988), pp. 1312-1313.

Martyn, C. N., D. J. Barker, C. Osmond, E. C. Harris, J. A.
Edwardson, and R. F. Lacey. "Geographical Relation
Between Alzheimer's Disease and Aluminum in Drinking
Water." *Lancet*, 1 (8629) (January 14, 1989), pp. 59-62.

McLachlan, D.R., W. J. Lukiw, and T. P. Kruck. "New Evidence
for and Active Roll of Aluminum in Alzheimer's Disease."
Canadian Journal of Neurological Sciences, 16 (4 Suppl)
(November, 1989), pp. 490-497.

Mindell, Earl R., Ph.D. *Unsafe at Any Meal.* New York:
Warner Books, 1987.

Moneret-Vautrin, D.A., G. Faure, and M. C. Bene. "Chewing-
Gum Preservative Induced Toxidermic Vasculitis." *Allergy*, 41 (September, 1986), pp. 546-548.

"More Than You Ever Thought You Would Know About Food
Additives." *FDA Consumer*, (February, 1982).

Mukherjee, Geeta Talukder and Archana Sharma. "Sister
Chromatid Exchanges Induced by Tertiary Butyl Hydro-
quinone in Bone Marrow Cells of Mice." *Environmental
and Molecular Mutagenesis*, 13 (1989), pp. 234-237.

Null, Gary. *The Complete Guide to Health and Nutrition.*
New York: Delacorte Press, 1984.

"Nutrition and Health." *The Surgeon General's Report*, U.S.
Department of Health and Human Services, Public Health
Service, DHS (PHS) Publication No. 88-50211. Washing-
ton, D.C.: 1988.

Ohshima, H., C. Furihata, T. Matsushima and H. Bartsch.
"Evidence of Potential Tumour-Initiating and Tumour-
Promoting Activities of Hickory Smoke Condensate When
Given Alone or With Nitrite to Rats." *Food and Chemical
Toxicology*, 27 (8) (August, 1989), pp. 511-516.

Pohl, Robert, M.D., Richard Balon, M.D., and Richard Ber-
chou, Phar. M.D. "Reaction to Chicken Nuggets in a
Patient Taking an MAOI." *American Journal of Psychi-
atry*, 145 (May, 1988), p. 651.

Prasad, Om and Gulshan Rai. "Haematological Abnormalities
Induced by Feeding a Common Artificial Sweetener,

Saccharin, in ICR Swiss Mice." *Toxicology Letters*, 36 (March, 1987), pp. 81-88.

Riggs, Betty S., M.D., Fred P. Harchelroad, Jr., M.D., and Cathy Poole, R.N. "Allergic Reaction to Sulfiting Agents." *Annals of Emergency Medicine*, Vol. 15 (January, 1986), pp. 77-79.

Sarkar, S., M. Nagabhushan, C. S. Soman, S. R. Tricker and S. V. Bhide. "Mutagenicity and Carcinogenicity of Smoked Meat from Nagaland, a Region of India Prone to a High Incidence of Nasopharyngeal Cancer." *Carcinogenesis*, 10 (4) (April, 1989), pp. 733-736.

Schauss, Alexander. *Diet, Crime and Delinquency*. Berkley, CA: Parker House, 1980.

Schwartz, George. *In Bad Taste: The MSG Syndrome*. Santa Fe, NM and San Francisco: Health Press, 1988.

Seeley, Lesley. "One Child's Poison." *Nursing Times*, 82 (29) (July 16-22, 1986), pp. 40-41.

Squire, E. N., Jr. "Angio-Oedema and Monosodium Glutamate." *Lancet*, 1 (April 25, 1987), p. 988.

Steinman, H. A., M.B., CH.B., D.C.H. and E. G. Weinberg, M.B., CH.B., F.C.P. "The Effects of Soft-Drink Preservatives on Asthmatic Children." *South African Medical Journal*, 70 (September 27, 1986), pp. 404-406.

Taffe, Bonita G. and Thomas W. Kensler. "Tumor Promotion by a Hydroperoxide Metabolite of Butylated Hydroxytoluene, 2,6-di-tert-Butyl-4-Hydroperoxy-4-Methyl-2, 5-Cyclohexadienone, in Mouse Skin." *Research Communications in Chemical Pathology and Pharmacology*, 61 (3) (September, 1988), pp. 291-303.

Taylor, Steve L., Ph.D., et al. "Sensitivity to Sulfited Foods Among Sulfite-Sensitive Subjects with Asthma." *Journal of Allergy and Clinical Immunology*, 81 (2) (June, 1988), pp. 1159-1167.

Thompson, David C. and Michael A. Trush. "Enhancement of Butylated Hydroxytoluene-Induced Mouse Lung Damage by Butylated Hydroxyanisole." *Toxicology and Applied Pharmacology*, 96 (1) (October, 1988), pp. 115-121.

Tsevat, Joel, M.D., Gary N. Gross, M.D., and Graeme P. Dowling, M.D. "Fatal Asthma After Ingestion of Sulfite-

Containing Wine." *Annals of Internal Medicine*, Vol. 170 (August, 1987), p. 263.

Walton, Ralph G., M.D. "Seizure and Mania After High Intake of Aspartame." *Psychosomatics*, 27 (March, 1986), pp. 218, 220.

Webb, Tony, Tim Lang, and Kathleen Tucker. *Food Irradiation, Who Wants It?* Rochester, Vermont, and Wellingborough, Northamptonshire: Thorsons Publishers, Inc., 1987.

Weiner, Michael A. *Bugs in the Peanut Butter*. Boston: Little, Brown & Co., 1976.

Winter, Arthur, M.D., and Ruth Winter. *Eat Right, Be Bright*. New York: St. Martin's Press, 1985.

Winter, Ruth. *A Consumer's Dictionary of Food Additives*. New York: Crown Publishers, Inc., 1989.

Wurtman, Richard J., M.D. "Aspartame: Possible Effect on Seizure Susceptibility." *Lancet*, 2 (November 9, 1985), p. 1060.

————. "Neurochemical Changes Following High-Dose Aspartame with Dietary Carbohydrates." *New England Journal of Medicine*, 309 (1983), pp. 429-430.

Wittenberg, Margaret M. *Experiencing Quality*. Austin, Texas: Whole Foods Market, 1987.

Zatta, P., R. Giordano, B. Corain, and G. G. Bombi. "Alzheimer Dementia and the Aluminum Hypothesis." *Medical Hypotheses*, 26 (2) (June, 1988), pp. 139-142.

Zukerman, L. Steven, M.D., et al. "Effect of Calcium-Binding Additives on Ventricular Fibrillation and Repolarization Changes During Coronary Angiography." *Journal of the American College of Cardiology*, 10 (December, 1987), pp. 1249-1253.

CHAPTER 2

FOODS WE SHOULD LIMIT

Cholesterol, fat, sodium and **sugar** are four components of foods that we, as a society, definitely need to limit. On the other hand, our bodies require some cholesterol, some fat and some salt to function properly. In addition, sugar is natural in all fruits so it can't be too bad. Unfortunately, our lifestyles have led us in a direction of overconsumption of these ingredients causing degenerative diseases such as heart disease, cancer, arthritis, hypertension, diabetes, etc., to take their toll.

Another sign of our times is **highly processed foods**. In most cases, nature gave us nutritious, well-balanced foods, but we, being the intelligent people that we are, figured we could go "one up" on nature. So we started changing foods by taking out what nature put in and replacing them with synthetic ingredients — more commonly referred to as additives and preservatives. In my opinion, these highly processed foods, together with our high fat consumption, are the biggest reasons why the American Cancer Society says that diet alone accounts for one third of all cancer deaths. The only reason this figure isn't much, much higher is that smoking and environmental hazards get us first. Have you ever thought about this? Even a person who smokes may live longer if he or she eats well.

In this chapter, we'll be discussing cholesterol, fat, sodium, sugar and highly processed foods, and we'll see why I recommend only limited consumption of foods containing higher than normal amounts of these ingredients.

CHOLESTEROL

Maybe the most talked about and least understood word in food today is cholesterol. Why? As a society, we just do not fully understand where and how our bodies get cholesterol. Everyone is saying that it's bad, and the manufacturers are having a heyday. Food products everywhere are adding "no cholesterol" signs to their labels. *Folks, 90% of these products with "no cholesterol" signs on them never had cholesterol in them anyway — never did — never will!* I actually think that a bicycle shop could hang a "no cholesterol" sign on their window and their sales would increase.

Let me share with you an experience I had a little over a year ago. I had been coming in contact with a number of people who, after discovering they had high cholesterol readings, were changing their diets in an effort to lower their cholesterol. The amazing thing I noticed was that the foods they were changing to actually were worse than what they were eating before. These people were trying to eat better, but were failing. Why was this happening?

Since I had been working with some health professionals in cholesterol testing, I approached them with this dilemma and suggested they work with me in an experiment. They agreed to my plan which randomly picked ten high cholesterol individuals. Each of these ten people were asked to go to their favorite grocery store and pick ten food products which they felt they should eat to help lower their cholesterol. Each person then brought the ten food products back to the testing sight so I could analyze the ingredients of each. They were so proud, and each thought he/she had really scored a winner. The results, however, were quite disappointing. On average, six out of the ten products purchased were very high in fat, and this is where the body gets most of its cholesterol.

Our bodies simply manufacture cholesterol from the fat we eat. Legally, a product can be 100% saturated fat and still say "no cholesterol" on the label. The *only* food products that contain cholesterol are animal products: all forms of meat — beef, liver, pork, chicken, fish, the yolk of all eggs, and all dairy products including cheese, milk, yogurt, cottage cheese, etc. Animal products can be very nutritious, but as a society, we are eating too many animal products for three reasons: too much fat, too much protein, and we get the cholesterol in the meat that the animal has already produced.

Just like us, animals produce cholesterol in the liver. Since cholesterol is a part of each cell (both in animals and people), the cholesterol that is in the meat products is passed on to us when we consume these products. But even though we receive cholesterol from animal products, most of the cholesterol we receive comes from the fat that we eat. I'm not talking just about animal fat either; I'm talking about animal and vegetable fat since we make cholesterol from both.

So, in essence, these people who were tested high in cholesterol wanted to make a change and were rushing to the grocery store and buying products which advertised "no cholesterol" and other health-related terms such as "all natural," but in reality, they were loaded with fat.

In another case, I saw a man with a blood cholesterol count of 240 milligrams (mg.). He decided to eliminate all animal products from his diet for two months. In other words, *he ate no cholesterol whatsoever for two months.* At the end of this time, he had his cholesterol checked again, and it was 280! An increase of 40 points, and he had eaten no cholesterol at all. His primary source of protein had been peanut butter, and his liver had done a dandy job of producing cholesterol from the plant fat in the peanut butter. In most cases, I believe that it's not so much the cholesterol we eat that causes high blood cholesterol, but rather the fat we eat.

Let's look at some traps we're apt to fall into while grocery shopping.

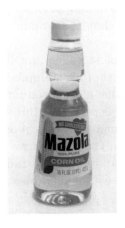

MAZOLA CORN OIL
"No Cholesterol"

Corn oil is produced from corn — a plant. Corn never had cholesterol in it and never will. However, corn oil is 100% fat. Every calorie in corn oil comes from fat.

SERVING	CALORIES	GRAMS OF FAT	% OF FAT
1 TB	120	14 g.	100%

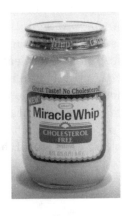

KRAFT MIRACLE WHIP
"Cholesterol Free"

Soybean oil is the primary ingredient in Miracle Whip, and soybean oil is 100% fat. As with all high-fat products, the use of this kind of spread needs to be limited for good health.

SERVING	CALORIES	GRAMS OF FAT	% OF FAT
1 TB	70	7 g.	90%

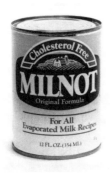

MILNOT EVAPORATED MILK
"Cholesterol Free"

Actually, this product has a small amount of cholesterol. The first ingredient is skim milk — an animal product. The law says though, that if the cholesterol is less than 2 mg. per 100 grams (g.), it can still be called cholesterol free. The cholesterol is not the culprit though; it's the fat — 48% of the calories come from fat, with the source being soybean oil.

SERVING	CALORIES	GRAMS OF FAT	% OF FAT
1/2 cup	150	8 g.	48%

As a society, we may consume too much protein-rich foods such as meat and dairy products. But, from a cholesterol standpoint, I feel that our fat consumption is the real culprit causing both degenerative heart disease and cancer as well as many other health problems.

The American Heart Association has recommended that a healthy adult should limit his/her cholesterol to 300 mg. per day. To be honest with you, I have never heard a good explanation for the 300 mg. figure. On the one hand, we don't even need to eat it; our bodies manufacture all we need. Yet, on the other hand, we are told that up to 300 mg. a day is okay. My problem is this: If we're overconsuming vegetable fat (no cholesterol in it), we're already going to get more cholesterol (via our liver) than our bodies need. In this case, even 5 mg. of additional cholesterol seems like too much to me.

To help you identify foods containing cholesterol, *The Food Bible* rates all foods containing any significant amount of cholesterol (20 mg. or more per serving) and will identify them.

FAT

What is fat? Webster says that fat is animal tissue consisting chiefly of cells distended with greasy or oily matter. Doesn't sound very appetizing, does it? But we need this greasy, oily matter. Fat helps give us shiny hair and a good complexion. Stored fat insulates us and helps keep our body temperature stabilized; it protects our organs from injury and provides us with energy.

I've been asked if there are any benefits to carrying around a little excess fat. Yes, there are a couple I can think of. It will keep us warmer in cold temperatures, and we could go longer without food than our skinny counterparts. The Chinese, for example, consume very little fat, and thus will not survive as long without food as most Americans. Of course, traditionally they have not had all the heart and cancer problems that we have either.

Fat is the most concentrated source of energy (calorie) in our diet. A gram of fat has nine calories; whereas a gram of protein or carbohydrate has four calories. In addition to supplying all this energy, fats carry the fat soluble vitamins A, D, E and K throughout our bodies.

Since we tend to overdo this good-tasting food, the American Heart Association has set a limit for healthy adults. They say that for good health we shouldn't get over 30% of our calories from fat. As we'll learn, knowing how much our bodies require is the easy part — figuring out if a food has fat in it and how much, can be a real task.

As a society, we are consuming between 40% and 60% of our calories from fat when 30% is recommended, but in my opinion, 20% would be even better. Remember, our bodies make cholesterol from the fat we eat. In fact, it is estimated that as much as 80%, and even more in some cases, of the cholesterol that accumulates in our bodies, comes directly from the fat we eat. But the cholesterol produced from fat is not the only problem resulting from fat. We are finding that excess fat also creates an ideal environment for cancer, heart disease, high blood pressure, and a host of other problems. I would have to rate our overconsumption of fat as the number one health concern in the United States. If fat is so bad, where is it coming from? Like one of my clients asked while trying to limit her fat consumption, "Why does everything I like have fat in it?" This is the exact response I get from anyone who has been overconsuming fat. We've heard about a "sweet tooth." Well, I feel that having a "fat tooth" is even more addictive. Once a person gets hooked on this taste, it is very addictive and all that person does is look for foods with the fatty taste. Let's look at a representative list of foods that are high in fat.

FOOD	% FAT	FOOD	% FAT
Coconut oil	100%	Salami	68%
Palm oil	100%	T-bone steak, lean & fat	68%
Margarine	100%	Ricotta cheese	67%
Mayonnaise	100%	Ground beef	66%
Cooking oils	100%	Potato chips, Pringles	64%
Coconut	92%	Parmesan cheese	62%
Cream cheese	90%	Candy bar, Mr. Goodbar	60%
Miracle Whip	90%	Cheesecake	58%
Pecans	90%	Mozzarella cheese	56%
Avocados	89%	Popcorn, Redenbacher's	56%
Salad dressing, French	86%	Ice cream, soft serve	55%
Almonds	82%	Tofu	53%
Frankfurter, beef	81%	Burger King fries	52%
Sunflower seeds, raw	79%	McDonald's Qtr. Pounder	51%
Bacon	76%	Croissant	50%
Peanut butter	76%	Milk, whole	48%
Pumpkin seeds	75%	Ice cream	47%
Cheddar cheese	70%	Cookies, chocolate chip	45%
Frankfurter, chicken	70%	T-bone steak, lean	44%

Any surprises? We are creatures of habit. I've known people who have moved to the United States from some third world countries where they were lucky if 10% of their diet was from fat. When confronted with our foods, they couldn't handle all the fat. The fat made them sick.

So, how does a person break a cycle of eating too much fat? The first step is to identify which foods are high in fat. *The Food Bible* will provide that link. The next step is up to

us. From experience in working with this problem, I generally recommend a gradual change. In fact, we could
become a "basket case" for a few days if we made the change
"cold turkey." A gradual change calls for replacing one high-
fat product we are now eating with a low-fat product. Once
our body has accepted this change, move on to another and
so on.

DILEMMA IN THE GROCERY STORE

We've decided that we want to start controlling our fat
intake; so now we head to the grocery store. As we begin to
look around for products low in fat, we find that the food
manufacturers have really been helpful. We see some cold
cuts that say *87% fat free*, so that goes in our basket. We also
see another that says *33% less fat*, and that must be good,
too, so that goes in our basket. Since we were thinking about
a salad, this *reduced calorie salad dressing* looks good, and
we put it in the basket. In just looking around for some
possible low-fat products, we find *Dream Whip* which says
"0" grams of fat, and we think, "Boy, I'll take two of those
home." Next we pick up a *healthful-looking granola cereal.*
We grab a loaf of *bread*, a head of *lettuce* for our salad, and
strawberries for that "0" fat Dream Whip and head home.
Once we're home we begin eating for a new lifestyle of
limited fat. To our surprise, we find that all these "low-fat"
foods taste really good, and we feel so excited that we have
made this change. *We have just done what literally thousands of people across the United States have done in hopes
for better health and renewed energy.*

Let's analyze what we purchased:

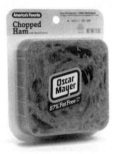

13% FAT?

OSCAR MAYER
87% FAT FREE

This 87% fat-free cold cut by Oscar Mayer is chopped ham. When we see only 13% fat, we assume that only 13% of the calories in the chopped ham come from fat, when in reality, **54%** of the calories are from fat. *Why*? In order to make a product look good, manufacturers list the percentage of fat by weight; whereas from a nutritional standpoint, fat should be measured by calories. So when we thought we were getting a nearly fat-free product, we ended up with one quite high in fat.

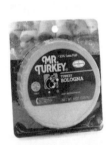

33% LESS FAT?

MR. TURKEY

This can really be confusing — 33% less fat than what? We really have no idea from this labeling what percentage of calories come from fat unless we do some figuring of our own. We have to look at the small print and get out our calculator. There are six grams of fat in each slice, and each slice has 70 calories. We take 6 x 9 (the number of calories in each gram of fat) and then divide by 70 (the calories in each slice).

$$6 \times 9 = 54 \div 70 = 77\%.$$

Now we see that this product gets **77%** of its calories from fat!

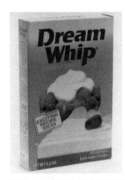

"0" GRAMS OF FAT?

DREAM WHIP

On the side of the box under nutrition, this product lists fat as "0" grams; yet the second ingredient is hydrogenated palm kernel oil, one of the highest saturated fat foods available. How can this be? The government says that a manufacturer can label a product as having "0" grams of fat as long as there is less than .5 grams of fat per serving. Dream Whip shows a serving size as one tablespoon, and one tablespoon has .33 grams of fat which is below the .5 gram limit; so the manufacturer can scratch out .33 and replace it with "0". In reality, this product has **45%** of its calories from fat, and we thought we were not getting any fat! Can you also imagine using only one level tablespoon of Dream Whip? Many times manufactureres intentionally lower serving sizes for this very reason — to make fat content look low, or as in this case, nonexistent. So this product that we bought two boxes of, actually is very high in fat when it appeared that it had no fat at all.

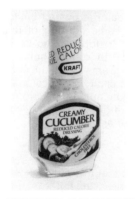

REDUCED CALORIES?

KRAFT CREAMY CUCUMBER REDUCED CALORIE SALAD DRESSING

Now for our salad, we purchased Kraft Creamy Cucumber dressing with reduced calories. Since it has only 25 calories per tablespoon, we really pour it on thick. But what the label doesn't tell us is that **72%** of those calories are from pure fat!

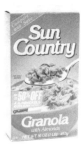

SUN COUNTRY GRANOLA

What about the cereal we bought for our breakfast? Actually we did pretty good here. It is nutritious and has ample fiber, but it is still a little high in fat — 35% of the calories come from fat, but considering that some of the fat is from nuts, that's about as good as we're going to do with that type food.

As I've stated, we must understand that the food industry is a very competitive business, and they use every trap they can to get us to buy. We like to blame them for false or misleading advertising, but in reality, it is we, the consumer, who dictates what a manufacturer produces. The manufacturer produces what we want, and the grocery stores stock what we will buy. So the choice is ours. We just need to become more educated about which foods are good for our health and which ones are not. If we start demanding the "good" foods, then that is what we will be seeing more of in our stores.

COOKING OILS

I am often asked which cooking oils are best to use. Personally, I prefer safflower oil; however, to understand why I rate this as number one, we need to look at the three different properties of oil. Remember though, all cooking oils are 100% fat and should be used very sparingly.

Three Properties of Oil:
Saturated . . . Monounsaturated . . . Polyunsaturated

Explaining the properties of oil can get quite technical if we don't have a chemistry background. For this reason, I'll use two approaches in explaining a subject that has, for the most part, been confusing. First, we'll use the "textbook" approach and then secondly, we'll use the "street language" approach.

Textbook Approach

Fats are really fatty acids made up of carbon, hydrogen and oxygen atoms. The differences in the saturation of fats lie in their molecular structure. Fats consist of carbon atoms linked together in a row. It is possible for each carbon atom to form bonds on all of its four sides, primarily with hydrogen and other carbon atoms. Sometimes a carbon atom will not link with a hydrogen atom, but instead it will form a double bond with the carbon atom next to it. If a molecule of fat lacks a hydrogen atom, it is called an *unsaturated fat*. If it has more than one double bond, or more open spaces, it is called *polyunsaturated*. (Poly means many.) If only one space is vacant, it is called a *monounsaturated fat*. (Mono means one.) If all the spaces are occupied with hydrogen atoms, it is called a *saturated fat*.

So, technically there are two classes of oils: saturated and unsaturated. However, the unsaturated has two distinguishing divisions, and these are monounsaturated and polyunsaturated. Mono, of course, meaning one, and poly more than one.

So, what does all this mean?

Street Language Approach

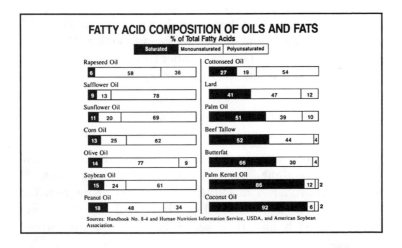

FATTY ACID COMPOSITION OF OILS AND FATS
% of Total Fatty Acids

| Saturated | Monounsaturated | Polyunsaturated |

Rapeseed Oil
6 | 58 | 36

Safflower Oil
9 13 | 78

Sunflower Oil
11 20 | 69

Corn Oil
13 25 | 62

Olive Oil
14 | 77 | 9

Soybean Oil
15 24 | 61

Peanut Oil
18 | 48 | 34

Cottonseed Oil
27 19 | 54

Lard
41 | 47 | 12

Palm Oil
51 | 39 | 10

Beef Tallow
52 | 44 | 4

Butterfat
66 | 30 | 4

Palm Kernel Oil
86 | 12 | 2

Coconut Oil
92 | 6 | 2

Sources: Handbook No. 8-4 and Human Nutrition Information Service, USDA, and American Soybean Association.

Remember, all fats contain some of each of these properties. The difference in oils is in the ratio of each of these properties to another. See chart. You'll see that rapeseed oil (canola) has the least amount of saturated fat and coconut oil has the most. You'll also see that olive oil is highest in monounsaturated and safflower oil is lowest and so on. If we were to take safflower oil (low in saturated and monounsaturated), olive oil (low in saturated and high in monounsaturated), and coconut oil (very highly saturated), and place a container of each on our kitchen table, we would see a distinct difference in texture.

safflower oil	It would be very runny.
olive oil	It would be thick but still runny.
coconut oil	It would be soft-solid and not run at all.

Now, take each of these oils and place them in your refrigerator for a while and see what happens.

safflower oil	It would still be runny.
olive oil	It would have become fairly solid.
coconut oil	It would have become a hard-solid.

This is the net result of what the textbook is telling us.

Highly saturated fats, such as coconut oil, lard, palm oils, butter, etc., are the firmer fats, and it is these type fats that are believed to be the primary contributors to the "bad" cholesterol that clogs our arteries.

Unsaturated fats such as safflower, soybean, corn, sunflower, etc., have often been given the identity of producing only "good" cholesterol. Whether this identity will hold up to the test of time remains to be seen. For example, the high monounsaturated property of olive oil is claimed by many health professionals to produce no "bad" cholesterol. Personally, I have a little trouble accepting this because these type oils turn solid at cool temperatures and are almost saturated. Most all health professionals, however, are in agreement that the saturated fats have more detrimental effects on our health than the unsaturated. This is why I will not include any food in *The Food Bible* that contains the highly saturated tropical fats: coconut, palm and palm kernel.

CAUTION

Let's look at a hypothetical situation. Let's say that a national health organization makes a public statement which says, "It has been determined that for good health we should avoid consumption of all saturated fats." The mistake we often make when reading a statement like this is that we assume that all other forms of fat have now been cleared, and we can consume all we want. *This is false and dangerous thinking.* Manufacturers will play on something like this, too. They'll start advertising "no saturated fats," and we, the public, will buy.

Folks, all forms of fat must be restricted not to exceed 30% of total calories consumed, and I feel that not over 20% would be even better. We just simply do not know for sure which types of fats contribute most to other conditions such as cancer, arthritis, stress, lack of energy, reduced nutrient absorption, diabetes, premature aging, etc. My best advice is to avoid saturated fats and limit all others — definitely not to exceed 30% of total calories consumed.

To help identify foods containing fat, *The Food Bible* rates all foods with over 30% of calories from fat as "high fat" and those foods with over 50% of calories from fat as "very high fat." In addition, foods containing the very highly saturated tropical fats and lard are not included in *The Food Bible.*

SODIUM

Another ingredient we Americans are getting way too much of is *sodium*. Like fat and cholesterol, our bodies require some sodium for good health, but here again, we have gone "crazy" with sodium, and it is showing in our health.

When we talk of sodium, we usually think of table salt. Table salt is made of sodium chloride, and we normally use it to flavor our foods. Sodium is an essential mineral which means that we must eat it — our body doesn't produce it. The majority of our bodies' sodium is in body fluids; within the blood vessels as well as within and around each and every cell. The remainder of the sodium is within the bones.

Sodium is a vital part of our electrolyte system which helps maintain the water balance as well as the pH balance of the body's fluids. An imbalance can lead to a heart attack and even death.

A high intake of sodium can also affect our blood pressure. Sodium attracts water. Since sodium is present primarily on the outside of the cells, it attracts extra water there and subsequently puts pressure on our blood vessels, causing high blood pressure or hypertension, and taxes the heart.

Since sodium is found virtually in all foods, it is rare to be deficient. What most of us Americans are concerned with is getting too much. In fact, the American Heart Association says that healthy adults should limit their sodium intake to around 3,000 mg. a day. How much is 3,000 mg.? Well, in the form of table salt, it's a little over one teaspoon. Keep in mind that we get sodium in practically all foods whether it's a glass of milk, a slice of bread or a carrot stick. So, when we eat a frozen dinner with 1,300 mg. of sodium, we're well on our way to our daily maximum with that one food product.

What's one man's castle is another man's cave. Throughout the course of time, salt has been a very valuable resource. In some civilizations it was even used as the equivalent of money. Only the very rich, generally the rulers, were allowed to use this valuable resource to enhance the taste of food. Sayings such as "the salt of the earth" developed as its symbolic goodness; both as value and taste. Haven't times changed? Today we're speaking of this very same salt as a burden. Oh, yes, it still tastes good, but that's the problem.

Nothing brings out the taste of food quite like salt, and manufacturers learned this trick years ago. They learned that they could take water, a little meat flavoring, meat broth, add salt (lots of it) and presto — they have a very tasty product! The fast food experts have also learned a trick of their own. As we know, they use an abundance of fat, and anytime a lot of fat is used in cooking, many of the natural flavors are lost. To compensate for this loss of taste, salt is added, and it is added unsparingly to create a flavor people will come back for. The hamburger and French fry market is what it is today because of two basic ingredients: fat and salt. In fact, the fast food market has had such an impact on food preferences (the fats and salts) that the grocery product manufacturers have had to change their recipes by adding more fat and salt just to stay competitive. I think a classic example of this is our soups. When Grandma used to prepare a soup for a friend with a cold, it had *health* written all over it. Now the word *caution* needs to be employed when buying most soups in the grocery store. Let's look at some popular brands:

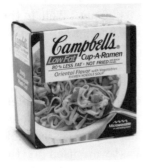

CAMPBELL'S LOW FAT CUP-A-RAMEN

One package (a serving) has 1,590 mg. of sodium and 180 calories. This is astronomically high in sodium. If we were to consume 1,800 calories in a day of this kind of food, we would have received 15,900 mg. of sodium. The American Heart Association says that 3,000 mg. a day is all we need, and here we get over half that amount in 180 calories.

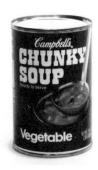

CAMPBELL'S CHUNKY VEGETABLE

One can, 10 3/4 ounces (a serving) has 1,100 mg. of sodium and 160 calories. Here again, this is very, very high in sodium. We get over one third of our sodium allotment in only 160 calories. Another way to look at sodium consumption: We shouldn't receive over 1.5 mg. of sodium per each calorie consumed. With Campbell's Chunky Vegetable Soup, we're getting 6.8 mg. of sodium per calorie consumed.

I'm not picking on Campbell's soup as most all brands of soup have this same pattern.

A trick that manufacturers sometime use to disguise the amount of sodium is with the serving size. Let's compare Weight Watchers cottage cheese with Borden cottage cheese:

	SERVING SIZE	CALORIES	SODIUM
W. W. cottage cheese	1 ounce	23	105 mg.
Borden cottage cheese	4 ounces	120	450 mg.

If we are comparing Weight Watchers with Borden, and we look only at the sodium content without checking the serving size, we would automatically think that Weight Watchers is four times lower in sodium. In reality, they are both fairly equal and both very high in sodium.

I have run experiments regarding food addictions and have found that when a diet of fat and salt become a regular part of one's eating pattern, this person actually begins to *crave* fried foods with lots of salt added. In order to reverse this lifestyle, a drying out period (as with any addiction) usually occurs. In conjunction with this drying out period, if a person substitutes healthful foods for the fat and salt, an amazing change occurs. In 30 to 90 days (the time varies), fatty and salty foods will actually *sound and taste repulsive.* It's very common to see a person go from "Please pass the salt" to "Please hold the salt."

All foods listed in *The Food Bible* are rated for sodium content, and those containing over 1.5 mg. of sodium per calorie are rated as "High Sodium" and those over 3.0 mg. of sodium per calorie are rated as "Very High Sodium."

SUGAR

The taste for sugar seems to be an innate characteristic of humans. I have seen newborn babies' reactions to different taste tests. They will screw up their faces and pucker at the sour and bitter tastes, but when given sugar-water, a look of pure pleasure comes over them — they almost smack their lips in joy! So, it seems that we're born with a liking for sweets.

Although it appears that our bodies can function without consuming any sugar, I feel that sugar is natural because it appears in so many of our natural foods such as fruits and milk. We have guidelines for cholesterol, fat and sodium consumption, but no one has really told us how much is too much sugar. Most just say we eat too much. The sugar from the fruits we eat is absorbed into our bodies along with the nutrients of the fruit. If we were a society that overconsumed fruit like we do fat, then we would probably see problems occur. We don't overconsume fruit, but we do one-up on nature and overconsume a very highly processed additive called *white sugar*. I call it an additive because it is not a food; it has absolutely no food value. All refined sugars are void of vitamins and minerals and have no fiber.

In addition, our bodies will absorb refined sugars into the bloodstream very quickly, causing a surge of energy plus a surge of insulin. Soon however, we experience a real "low" or fatigue brought about by the excess insulin production. The natural unrefined sugars in fruits, milk, etc. are absorbed at a controlled steady rate so there is not the extreme sudden rise in our blood sugar level that we have with any of the refined sugars. Think of this: Sugar cane (one source of white sugar) in its natural state has fiber, vitamins, minerals, amino acids, trace elements and is *16% to 20% sucrose*. After sugar cane has been processed into white sugar, it has been stripped of everything, leaving a substance with *99% pure sucrose*. It's the eating of this type sugar that puts so much stress on our bodies.

We find refined sugar in our food products listed a variety of ways: brown sugar, powdered sugar, honey, molasses, maple sugar, corn syrup, corn syrup solids, sorghum, etc. I have seen many people who think they are buying a product without sugar because the word *sugar* was not listed as one of the ingredients. I think a classic example is ketchup.

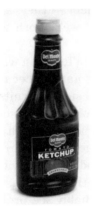

KETCHUP

Ketchup is high in sugar, but the word *sugar* doesn't appear in the ingredients. Concentrated corn syrup, used in this ketchup, is much higher in calories per unit than white sugar.

Health professionals are not in complete agreement on the damage that the overconsumption of sugar can do to our bodies. I believe that the hyperactivity we're seeing in many of our children today is partially the result of too much sugar as well as the additives and preservatives which many times accompany high sugar products. Some health professionals disagree, but I don't buy it. I have had too many clients with hyperactive children who have told me that when sugar consumption is reduced, their hyperactivity decreases. So what about adults? I think the same rule applies. We adults have just learned to control our actions somewhat.

Keep this in mind though, each person has a different sugar tolerance level, and what is too much for one person may be within another person's limits. Is some diabetes, high blood sugar levels, etc. the result of eating too much sugar for too many years? Like I said, health professionals are not in agreement, but they *are* in agreement that if we have diabetes or high blood sugar levels, we certainly should reduce sugar consumption. Sounds like the old adage, "which came first, the chicken or the egg." I have one firm conviction — don't overconsume refined sugar.

On the other side of the coin, I would like to defend sugar. Most people blame sugar and sugar products for weight problems. Sure, sugar plays a role, but for most of us, the real culprit is fat. Let me be more specific. A teaspoon of white sugar has approximately 16 calories; whereas a teaspoon of fat has approximately 40 calories! Let's look at an example:

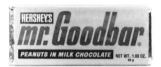

MR. GOODBAR

This candy bar has 270 calories: 30% or 80 calories come from sugar; 60% or 162 calories come from fat; 10% or 27 calories come from other carbohydrates and protein.

SUMMARY

I have absolutely no problem with the sugar we receive in whole foods such as fruits. They're natural, they are nutritious, and they provide fiber. My real concern is with the highly processed sugars such as white sugar, corn syrup, brown sugar, etc., and yes, even honey. In my opinion, these type sugars that get into our bloodstream so quickly causing insulin surges, hyperactivity, etc. are what we should be most concerned about. Many times these sugars are hidden in our grocery products. We just need to know which ones they are and make an effort to limit their use. *The Food Bible* identifies those products high in refined sugars.

HIGHLY PROCESSED FOODS

Processed foods are a product of our society. As consumers, we demand foods that taste good, look good, have a long shelf life and are convenient and easy to prepare. The convenient and easy to prepare concept is the grocery store's answer to the fast food restaurant industry. If we can't grab a ready-prepared meal from our freezer or cupboard, throw it in the microwave and be eating it within five minutes, we'll probably look for something a little quicker the next time we visit the grocery store. We are a very time conscious society. The food industry realizes this, and each manufacturer is competing with the other to make their food quicker and easier to prepare plus taste and look like a gourmet meal made from "scratch."

Two things almost always occur during food processing. First, some of the *natural* food properties are taken out; and secondly, some *unnatural* food properties are added. There are some exceptions such as pure orange juice where only food properties are taken out, but let's take a look at the very best form of orange juice — not the ones where sugars and other ingredients have been added. On average we would have to squeeze approximately five oranges to produce one cup of orange juice. Let's compare the nutrients of five oranges with one cup of orange juice.

NUTRIENT	FIVE ORANGES	ONE CUP ORANGE JUICE
Vitamin C	400 mg.	124 mg.
Folacin	235 mg.	109 mg.
Calcium	280 mg.	27 mg.
Vitamin A	125 RE	50 RE
Potassium	1,250 mg.	496 mg.
Fiber	8.9 g.	.75 g.

mg. = milligram   R E = Retinol Equivalent   g. = gram

Orange juice is very nutritious, but look at all the nutrients we throw away in the pulp. Almost all the fiber and calcium are lost, and the other nutrients listed are greatly reduced. Compared to the processing that many of our foods go through, orange juice is not generally thought of as a processed food.

Let's look at another simple form of processing — that of converting peanuts to peanut oil. Peanuts, although very high in fat, are quite nutritious. However, when processed into peanut oil, the only thing the oil has left in it is *VITAMIN E, FAT, AND CALORIES.* **All the other nutrients and all the fiber are lost in processing.**

These are only simple forms of processing. Think what happens with some of the very highly processed food products such as some of our cereals, breads, rice, frozen and packaged dinners, etc. In fact, in many cases, nutrients have to be added back in (enriched) just so it can be called food. Sometimes I think that we could eat a bowl of sawdust, doctor it up to taste good, add a "one-a-day" vitamin, and we could receive the same benefit. Somehow, I feel that our bodies can tell the difference!

To realize that many additives are a part of our foods, all we have to do is look at the long list under ingredients on each label. Most of the words we can't even pronounce, let alone know what they mean. Let's look at two boxed pasta meals and compare their ingredients.

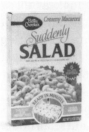   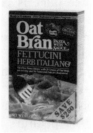

**Betty Crocker
Suddenly Salad
Creamy Macaroni**

INGREDIENTS:
enriched macaroni
dried peas
dried carrots
modified corn starch
sugar
salt
maltodextrin
spice
vinegar
MSG*
paprika
dried garlic
dried onion
natural flavors
whey
citric acid
partially hydrogenated
    soybean oil
disodium inosinate*
disodium guanylate*
color & freshness
preserved by:
    sodium sulfite*
    sodium bisulfite*
BHA*

**Health Valley
Oat Bran
Pasta & Sauce**

INGREDIENTS:
oat bran
whole wheat flour
brown rice flour
corn flour
soy flour
spices:
    tomato powder
    marjoram
    thyme
    oregano
    rosemary
    savory
    sage
    sweet basil
    sea salt
    onion powder
    garlic powder

The product on the left didn't even get into *The Food Bible*. I have asterisked the reasons why, plus the main ingredient in the macaroni is very highly processed.

The product on the right not only got in *The Food Bible*, but it also received the "Star Rating." All ingredients are unprocessed and natural, and all flavorings are provided by natural spices.

Many nutritionists and manufacturers claim that by enriching a highly processed food, we get back what was lost. No way . . . not even close. The nutrient level of the product on the right is much superior to the enriched one on the left. Plus it appears that the manufacturer of the product on the left is so ashamed of the lack of fiber that they didn't even list it on the box. The product on the right has ten grams of dietary fiber per nine-ounce serving.

We, the consumers, are partly responsible for this because we demand foods to *taste good, look good, have a long shelf life, and to be convenient and easy to prepare.* Each manufacturer is competing for our business, and all of them are using every legal method available to get us to buy their products. Let's explore!

Foods Must Taste Good

Fat, salt, sugar, NutraSweet, saccharin, monosodium glutamate, disodium guanylate, disodium inosinate, and artificial flavorings have become very common ingredients added to foods just for taste. We have become hooked on these tastes. We demand these tastes, and we're paying the price.

Foods Must Look Good

Food coloring, alginic acid, BHA, BHT, EDTA, silicon dioxide and sulfites are a few ingredients added to foods to make them look fresh and brightly colored. I know of farmers who really chuckle when they see the foods in a grocery store that they have grown. What they're chuckling about is that we consumers think that all those bright colors, such as bright green broccoli and peas, are natural and a sign of freshness.

Many times EDTA is added to remove zinc and other valuable minerals from such foods as frozen peas to make them appear a bright color. Manufacturers also know that children are attracted to bright colors, and thus we're seeing bright-colored cereals, Kool-Aid, Jell-O, fruit snacks, etc. Yes, and we, the consumer, are paying the price both out of our pockets and with our health.

Foods Must Have A Long Shelf Life

This is really where the term preservative takes on meaning. Grandma and our ancestors had their own tricks to preserve food. They used salt on meat; they sun dried fruits and meats; they canned meats, fruits and vegetables; they buried potatoes in the oat bin, and they hung onions in the hayloft to dry. Today we're more sophisticated. We don't use the hayloft and oat bin anymore, but we still use canning and salt, plus refrigeration and freezing in addition to a number of preservatives to keep foods from spoiling.

I am sympathetic to the food industry in this area. If we let foods spoil and then eat them, we have problems; and yet, when eating foods with certain preservatives, we have problems. It's just a matter of knowing which are the best choices. In my opinion, refrigeration and freezing rank right at the top.

Foods Must Be Convenient
And Easy To Prepare

A few years back when I used to teach cooking and food preparation classes, one of my main goals was to have a meal on the table in fifteen minutes. I'm all for convenience; however, one convenience really has me concerned. This is our cured meats such as bologna, salami, ham, frankfurters, etc. These foods are cured with nitrites which, in my opinion, are very dangerous when consumed over a period of time.

I haven't seen any recent figures, but it wouldn't surprise me to see nitrite-cured meat consumption, for many people, equal to or exceeding fresh meat consumption. Nitrite-cured meats are those with the pink color such as cured hams, frankfurters, etc. Oh, yes, the pepperoni on that delicious pizza is nitrite-cured, too — what a shame!

FIBER

The one common thread that I see in most all processing is the loss of dietary fiber. Everyone seems to know quite a few foods that contain fiber and most everyone knows that there is something good about fiber, but I find that few understand what fiber really is. Some of this misunderstanding is justified because the rules keep changing. Put more succinctly, we're learning new ways to measure fiber, and we're still learning what all its benefits include. There are even conflicting beliefs about whether too much can be harmful.

First, let's define fiber. *Fiber is simply that part of plant foods which our bodies do not digest.* Animal foods do not contain fiber. Certain natural plant foods are simply designed so that parts of that food will pass on through our bodies, acting as a cleansing or purifying agent. Our bodies receive toxins in many of the foods we eat, and it is these undigested food parts (fiber) that help remove some of these toxins. Of course, we also have our liver, spleen, etc., and the entire immune system standing ready to attack any foreign agent that didn't get flushed out.

As I see it, research is at a point today where we know for sure that fiber is good. We know that it is needed for good health, and we know some specific benefits that it provides. What we're still learning is exactly how many benefits fiber has, what they are, and if too much is damaging. Food manufacturers have really used fiber well in promoting their products. It kind of amuses me — they process a food and take out most of the natural fiber, then advertise that fiber has been added, and it really sells — a la some of our cereals!

How Is Fiber Measured?

Pick up two different reference guides and you'll likely see two different types of measurements — *crude fiber and dietary fiber*. Why? Crude fiber employs an older method of measurement where strong chemicals are used to digest food. What is left undigested is called crude fiber. The dietary fiber measurement employs the use of milder chemicals and enzymes. The undigested food parts remaining in this approach is called dietary fiber.

Scientists feel that the dietary measurement more closely

resembles our bodies, so the complete system of measuring fiber is being converted to the dietary fiber approach. There are two reasons why we're still seeing crude fiber measurements listed. The first being that some people resist change and are still using the old rules; and secondly, all foods simply have not yet been accurately measured for dietary fiber. Although foods will vary, we have been given an approximate conversion formula which is: crude fiber $\times$ 3 = dietary fiber.

Even this new approach of measuring fiber is not an exact science, and at best, we can only arrive at approximate measurements. In addition, each person's digestive system will vary, causing additional deviations. The bottom line, though, is that we have a good system for measuring approximate dietary fiber in plant foods.

IS THERE MORE THAN ONE KIND OF FIBER?

Yes. *Soluble Fiber* **and** *Insoluble Fiber.*

Soluble Fiber

Soluble fiber's most distinctive characteristic is that this form of fiber absorbs water, as well as other substances, and is easily fermented while traveling through the digestive tract. Think of it as a legion of mini-sponges traveling through our bodies. Foods that are high in soluble fibers include citrus fruits, apples, legumes, carrots, barley, oatmeal, oat bran and so on.

Research is uncovering some very interesting traits of soluble fiber. These fibers are believed to help lower blood cholesterol, regulate blood sugar levels and absorb and remove toxins and carcinogens from our bodies. Scientists are not quite sure how these feats are all performed, but evidence certainly shows that it is happening. Somehow these little sponge-like particles of certain foods collect and discard properties, that if left in our bodies, may cause problems.

Sounds great to me, but let's look at a scary scenario. Let's assume that we're eating a lot of fat and cholesterol products, a lot of additives and preservatives, and not eating foods rich in soluble fiber — the very foods that tend to forgive us for overconsumption of the enemies. It certainly isn't very hard for me to understand why the American Cancer Society is now saying that the leading cause of cancer in the United States is due to the foods we are eating; and I guess, not eating in this case.

Soluble fiber also has a side benefit. Since it swells as it passes through our bodies, it gives us a feeling of fullness and helps curb overeating. Try it sometime. Compare eating a serving of oatmeal (high in soluble fiber) and a serving of Grape Nuts (high in insoluble fiber) and see which gives you a more full feeling.

Insoluble Fiber

Insoluble fiber is that fiber which passes through our bodies in essentially the same form it entered. Foods that are high in insoluble fiber include wheat bran, whole wheat breads and cereals, leafy vegetables and some fruits and nuts. These foods will also have some soluble fiber, but they are predominately insoluble and are generally categorized as such.

Insoluble fiber features the acceleration of food through our bodies, especially in the small and large intestines. Insoluble fiber has been recommended to increase the bulk of our stool and to lower the risk of colon cancer. The reasoning is that this type fiber hurries digested foods through our intestines faster, lessening the chance for infection and irritation of the colon. Also, if carcinogens are present, they will exit the body more rapidly (if they haven't already been absorbed), thus lessening the chance for cancer.

Can We Get Too Much?

The National Cancer Institute recommends that we receive between *20 to 30 grams of dietary fiber per day*. Other experts recommend between 20 and 45 grams per day. The fact is, we do not know for sure how much is needed. All experts are in agreement though, that our current average fiber consumption of between 10 and 15 grams per day is far too low.

But, can we get too much? Yes and no. At least that's what we're hearing. Some health professionals feel that too much fiber, especially the insoluble form, will cause mineral depletion. Their thinking is that this form of fiber increases the speed at which food travels through our bodies, so some minerals do not have time to be absorbed.

Others say that the very foods that are high in insoluble fiber are also high in mineral content, so this in itself will offset any loss. There is even a recent study from the University of Maryland suggesting that insoluble fiber actually helps with the absorption of minerals. While the professionals are doing their testing, I feel we can do a little self-examination of our own.

If we haven't been eating a lot of fiber-rich foods and suddenly decide to go to 30 or 40 grams per day, we will probably find ourselves in the bathroom fairly often. To me this means we're getting too much. It takes our bodies time to adjust to changes, so it is best to gradually increase fiber intake until we get in the 25 to 35 gram range. Our bodies will tell us how much we can handle.

The balance between soluble and insoluble fiber and their unique roles in helping our bodies to cleanse is very interesting and fascinating. If we're eating the kinds of foods we know we should, we'll automatically get our required fiber intake. To get enough fiber, just think —

- 50% to 60% of our calories from *complex carbohydrates* which include whole grains such as: wheat, oats, rye, barley, rice, etc.; and starchy vegetables such as: potatoes, corn, peas, winter squash, legumes, etc.
- 25% to 30% of our calories from *simple carbohydrates* which include all fruits such as: apples, oranges, bananas, etc.; and vegetables such as: carrots, tomatoes, onions, cabbage, broccoli, etc.

SUMMARY

Highly processed foods, in many respects, deliver a "double whammy." On the one hand, valuable nutrients and fiber are taken out, leaving, at best, a food look-alike; on the other hand, artificial ingredients have been added back, that in themselves, are counterproductive.

On the bright side, I am seeing a few smaller food companies trying to reverse this trend. These are companies which are manufacturing wholesome, limited processed foods without any of the dangerous additives and preservatives. They are offering some very outstanding choices for us, the consumer. Most are distributed nationally, and if these products are not already on our shelves, most grocery stores will add them if the demand is there. We just have to ask. Grocery stores will stock their shelves with what we want. If we demand and purchase the highly processed (the fats, etc.), then that is what will be offered.

However, if we demand and purchase the good foods, then that is what will be offered. Change does take time, but I do see it coming. We just need to be persistent. Know what we want and ask for it. It is our right.

All foods listed in *The Food Bible* which are highly processed are identified and rated as such.

CHAPTER 3

HOW FOODS ARE RATED

We have talked about the three basic categories of foods.

Category I Foods (those found to have ingredients in them that we should avoid) have **not** been included in *The Food Bible*. I simply rated their risk too great to include them in *The Food Bible*.

Category II Foods (those that have ingredients in them that we should limit) are included in *The Food Bible* and are identified and rated. These are foods which contain high levels of fat, sodium and refined sugars; foods that are highly processed; and foods containing significant amounts of cholesterol.

Category III Foods (those that do not appear to have any use-limitations) are included in *The Food Bible* and are given the Star (★) Rating.

HOW GROCERY PRODUCTS ARE
CODED IN *THE FOOD BIBLE*

To save space and to make *The Food Bible* as easy to use as possible, I have designed a very simple coding system. The system works as follows:

The number (1) = High Fat

The number (2) = High Sodium

The number (3) = High Refined Sugar

The number (4) = Highly Processed

The number (5) = High Cholesterol

The Star (★) = Does not include any of the above.

Now, let's explore each rating to fully understand its purpose in making food selections.

FAT

The American Heart Association recommends that the diet of a healthy adult should not exceed 30% of its calories from fat. If we purchase a frozen dinner that has 320 calories and 14 grams of fat per serving, we need to do some calculating to find the percentage of calories from fat. Since each gram of fat has nine calories, let's take this information and figure out the percentage of calories from fat.

Take the grams of fat per serving (14) times the calories per gram (9). Divide the calories from fat (126) by the calories per serving (320). This figure gives us the percentage of calories from fat.

$$14 \times 9 = 126 \text{ calories from fat}$$

$$126 \div 320 = .39 \text{ or } 39\% \text{ of calories from fat}$$

This frozen dinner, Cheese Manicotti by Weight Watchers, gets 39% of its calories from fat — definitely higher than what is recommended for good health.

So, using this measurement as a guide, any food product listed in *The Food Bible* that derives over 30% of its calories from fat is rated "High Fat" and is given a rating code of (1).

Since there are so many products which contain *very* high levels of fat, I believe that these need to be specifically identified. Therefore, any product which contains over 50% of its calories from fat is rated "Very High Fat" and is given a rating code of (1+). As an example: The Kraft frozen dinner, Sirloin Chili Size with Steak Fries has 380 calories and 22 grams of fat. It gets 52% of its calories from fat and is given a rating code of (1+).

If a product does not have a 1 or 1+ rating, this means that less than 30% of its calories comes from fat. If you are watching your fat intake, these foods, of course, will be your best choices.

SUMMARY OF RATING CODES FOR FAT

(1) = High Fat (30%-50% of calories from fat)

(1+) = Very High Fat (over 50% of calories from fat)

Foods without a 1 or 1+ have less than 30% of their calories from fat and are your best choices.

SODIUM

The American Heart Association recommends that the daily sodium intake for a healthy adult be limited to around 3,000 mg. per day. So, using this measurement as a guide and using an average of 2,000 calories consumed per day, we can arrive at a guideline for maximum recommended sodium intake. For every calorie consumed, we should not receive over 1.5 mg. of sodium; in other words, a 1 to 1.5 ratio. As an example: If you purchase a can of Health Valley Lentil Soup that has 170 calories and 435 mg. of sodium per serving, you divide the sodium (435) by the calories (170).

$$435 \div 170 = 2.6 \text{ mg. of sodium per calorie}$$

This means that for every calorie in this can of soup, there are 2.6 mg. of sodium. Since this exceeds the recommended maximum of 1.5 mg. of sodium to 1 calorie, this product is high in sodium and is given a rating code of (2).

This computation may seem a bit confusing, but be assured, I have computed the sodium content for all products in *The Food Bible*. Any product with more than 1.5 mg. sodium per calorie is rated "High Sodium" and is given a rating code of (2).

As with fat, many products have exceedingly high levels of sodium, and I feel that these need to be identified separately. As an example: A can of Hain's New England Clam Chowder has 180 calories and 780 mg. of sodium per serving, or 4.3 mg. of sodium per calorie. This means that for every calorie in this can of soup, there are 4.3 mg. of sodium.

Any product over 3.0 mg. of sodium per calorie is rated "Very High Sodium" and is given a rating code of (2+).

If a product does not have a 2 or 2+ rating, this

means that the sodium content is under the 3,000 mg. maximum recommended for good health. And if you are watching your sodium intake, these foods, of course, will be your best choices.

SUMMARY OF RATING CODES FOR SODIUM

(2) = High Sodium (in excess of 1.5 mg. sodium per calorie)

(2+) = Very High Sodium (in excess of 3.0 mg. sodium per calorie)

Foods without a 2 or 2+ rating have less than 1.5 mg. sodium per calorie and are your best choices.

SUGAR

No guidelines have been established for maximum sugar intake. However, the American Diabetic Association and many other health professionals agree that the more highly processed types of sugar, those that enter the bloodstream very quickly, should be limited. I have identified these foods in *The Food Bible* which contain high amounts of refined sugars. They are rated "High Sugar" and have a rating code of (3).

Keep in mind that such foods as fruits and dairy products are naturally sweet. Any products that have been sweetened with natural fruit juices — not refined sugars — will not be given a rating code. The purpose of this rating is to identify only those foods which contain a significant amount of refined sugars.

If a product does not have a 3 rating, this means that it does not contain a high level of refined sugar. These foods will be your best choices.

SUMMARY OF RATING CODE FOR SUGAR

(3) = High Refined Sugar

Foods without a 3 rating do not contain high levels of refined sugars. If you are concerned with your refined sugar intake, these foods are your best choices.

HIGHLY PROCESSED

Highly processed foods are characterized by reduced nutrients and substantially reduced fiber content. Many health professionals now believe that our low fiber intake in the United States has been associated with some types of cancers, and some fibers are believed to help reduce cholesterol. To help identify foods listed in *The Food Bible* that are highly processed, I have rated these foods as "Highly Processed" and have given them a rating code of (4).

If a product does not have a 4 rating, this means that it is not highly processed. If you are concerned about selecting foods which still contain most of their natural nutrients and fiber, these foods are your best choices.

SUMMARY OF RATING CODE FOR
HIGHLY PROCESSED FOODS

(4) = Highly Processed

Foods without a 4 rating have more natural nutrients and fiber and are the best choices if you want to avoid highly processed foods.

CHOLESTEROL

The cholesterol rating is designed to identify foods listed in *The Food Bible* which contain a significant amount of cholesterol. I have identified a significant amount as 20 mg. or more per serving. So, using this as a guideline, any product in *The Food Bible* which contains 20 mg. or more of cholesterol per serving is rated "Cholesterol" and is given the rating code of (5).

If a product does not have a 5 rating, this means that it

has fewer than 20 mg. of cholesterol per serving. If you are watching your cholesterol intake, these products, of course, are your best choices.

SUMMARY OF RATING CODE FOR CHOLESTEROL

(5) = Cholesterol (20 mg. or more per serving)

Foods without a 5 rating have fewer than 20 mg. cholesterol per serving. If you are watching your cholesterol intake, these foods are your best choices.

STAR RATING

If you are concerned about eating foods that are not high in fat, not high in sodium, not high in refined sugars, not highly processed, and ones that do not contain a significant amount of cholesterol, then all "Star-Rated" foods will be your best choices. *The Food Bible* clearly identifies all Star-Rated foods with a (★).

CAUTION: Please understand that our bodies require fat, sodium, and cholesterol to function properly. It is only the overconsumption of products containing high levels of fat, sodium, and cholesterol that can be dangerous. For this reason, do not assume that only Star-Rated foods are nutritious foods. For example: The almond is very high in fat but is also very nutritious. The almond does not receive the Star-Rating because of this one limitation, but that does not make it less nutritious.

So, when you are using *The Food Bible*, do not automatically assume that all Star-Rated foods are good and all the others are bad. There are many foods with rating codes of (1), (2), (3) and (5) which are very nutritious, but consumption should be limited or controlled. However, I personally do not consider any food with a rating code of (4) to be very nutritious.

FOOD PRODUCTS *NOT* INCLUDED
IN *THE FOOD BIBLE*

(1) Any food products that I found to contain one or more of the ingredients listed in Chapter 1 **will not** be included in *The Food Bible*. These are foods which I feel should be avoided as much as possible because of their potentially dangerous ingredients. Therefore, you will not find any of these foods listed in *The Food Bible*. I simply deemed them not good enough to make *The Food Bible*.

(2) For the most part, local products **will not** be included in *The Food Bible*. Dairy products often fall into this category. There are many very fine local products, but they are not included for obvious reasons — a person in Atlanta is not interested in foods offered only in California.

I have tried very hard to include and rate all national and regional brands. I am in constant contact with grocery stores, food distributors, and food manufacturers so that I may be aware of most all products offered. But keep in mind, there are many thousands of food products offered with many changing their ingredients quite regularly. In addition, we have new products that are constantly arriving on our grocery shelves. I guess what I'm saying is that as hard as I try to include all products, I will miss some.

CHAPTER 4

INTRODUCTION TO RATED FOODS

Dear Reader,

As you begin using *The Food Bible*, I'm sure you will notice that certain companies keep appearing at the top of the ratings. In addition to some very fine products offered by larger companies, there are smaller companies that are really making a strong effort to put very healthful products on our grocery shelves. Some of these companies include:

Health Valley	R. W. Knudsen	Fantastic Foods
Arrowhead Mills	Barbara's	New Morning
Hodgson Mill	Hain	Natures Warehouse

Because of these companies' sizes, I have observed that they are not yet included in all grocery stores. However, this does not mean that a grocery store can't get them. We just need to let our grocer know that we want these products and ask the manager to please include these items.

If for any reason you have problems getting the selections you want in your area, please let me know. I am in contact with most manufacturers and would be glad to help from this end. Please direct any questions or concerns to:

PRS
Box 1828
Edmond, OK 73083-1828

PLEASE NOTE:

As an aid to *The Food Bible*, I strongly encourage you to consider **The Food Bible Companion**, a monthly newsletter. Like bread and butter, *The Food Bible* and **The Companion** generally work best together. Details for ordering are provided at the end of this book on page 363.

Jayne Benkendorf

TABLE OF CONTENTS FOR ALL FOODS

84

As an additional aid in locating specific foods, see "Food Index" beginning on page 355.

LISTING OF
ALL FOODS

BABY FOODS

Most baby foods are free of additives and preservatives. There are a few exceptions such as:

Gerber Zwieback Toast	potassium bromate
Heinz Barley Cereal	cottonseed oil

In addition to the additives and preservatives, I find that most mothers are concerned about their infants eating refined sugar. Baby food that contains refined sugar has a rating code of (3). Refined sugars are found most frequently in infant fruits and fruit desserts. Fruits contain sugar naturally, and it is not necessary to add refined sugar, which has no nutrients or fiber, and replaces fruit, which does have nutrients and fiber.

Many infant dinners contain refined pasta and rice. Personally, I would purchase a vegetable and meat infant dinner, then add my own whole wheat pasta or brown rice. This will add many valuable nutrients which were destroyed in the processing of the refined pasta and rice.

As for juices, I would give infants the same juices I drink — unless they must be strained for bottle feeding.

Most all baby formulas contain coconut oil. After talking with baby formula companies, I understand that coconut oil is necessary to make the formulas as close to mother's milk as possible. Since I do not include food or drink in *The Food Bible* that contains coconut oil, I am not listing baby formulas.

Since most people purchase baby food by brands, this is the way I have listed them.

VARIETY (Brand)   RATING CODE

VARIETY (Brand)	Fat	Sodium	Sugar	Processed	Cholesterol	Better Choice
BABY FOOD						
BEECH-NUT						
BABY'S FIRST						
Applesauce *(Beech-Nut)*						★
Bananas *(Beech-Nut)*						★
Carrots *(Beech-Nut)*		2				
Peaches *(Beech-Nut)*						★
Pears *(Beech-Nut)*						★
Peas *(Beech-Nut)*						★
Squash *(Beech-Nut)*						★
Sweet Potatoes *(Beech-Nut)*						★
STAGE 1						
Applesauce *(Beech-Nut)*						★
Bananas *(Beech-Nut)*						★
Barley Cereal *(Beech-Nut)*						★
Beef & Beef Broth *(Beech-Nut)*	1				5	
Carrots *(Beech-Nut)*		2+				
Chicken & Chicken Broth *(Beech-Nut)*	1				5	
Green Beans *(Beech-Nut)*						★
Lamb & Lamb Broth *(Beech-Nut)*	1				5	
Oatmeal Cereal *(Beech-Nut)*				4		
Peaches *(Beech-Nut)*						★
Pears *(Beech-Nut)*						★
Peas *(Beech-Nut)*						★
Rice Cereal *(Beech-Nut)*				4		
Squash *(Beech-Nut)*						★
Sweet Potatoes *(Beech-Nut)*						★
Turkey & Turkey Broth *(Beech-Nut)*	1+				5	
Veal & Veal Broth *(Beech-Nut)*						★
STAGE 2						
Apples & Strawberries Supreme Dessert *(Beech-Nut)*			3			
Apples, Peaches & Strawberries Supreme Dessert *(Beech-Nut)*			3			
Apples, Pears & Bananas Supreme Dessert *(Beech-Nut)*			3			

1 = High Fat   2 = High Sodium   3 = High Refined Sugar   5 = Cholesterol
1+ = Very High Fat   2+ = Very High Sodium   4 = Highly Processed   ★= Better Choice

VARIETY *(Brand)*   RATING CODE

Variety (Brand)	★	1	3	4
Applesauce & Apricots *(Beech-Nut)*	★			
Applesauce & Bananas *(Beech-Nut)*	★			
Applesauce & Cherries *(Beech-Nut)*	★			
Apricots with Pears & Applesauce *(Beech-Nut)*	★			
Banana Pineapple Dessert *(Beech-Nut)*			3	
Bananas & Yogurt *(Beech-Nut)*			3	
Bananas with Pears & Applesauce *(Beech-Nut)*	★			
Beef & Egg Noodle Dinner with Vegetables *(Beech-Nut)*		1		
Beef Dinner Supreme *(Beech-Nut)*		1		
Chicken & Rice Dinner with Vegetables *(Beech-Nut)*		1		
Chicken Noodle Dinner with Vegetables *(Beech-Nut)*	★			
Cottage Cheese with Pineapple *(Beech-Nut)*			3	
Creamed Corn *(Beech-Nut)*	★			
Dutch Apple Dessert *(Beech-Nut)*			3	
Fruit Dessert *(Beech-Nut)*	★			
Garden Vegetables *(Beech-Nut)*	★			
Guava Tropical Fruit Dessert *(Beech-Nut)*			3	
Macaroni & Beef Dinner *(Beech-Nut)*		1		
Mango Tropical Fruit Dessert *(Beech-Nut)*			3	
Mixed Cereal *(Beech-Nut)*				4
Mixed Cereal with Applesauce & Bananas *(Beech-Nut)*				4
Mixed Fruit & Yogurt *(Beech-Nut)*			3	
Mixed Vegetables *(Beech-Nut)*	★			
Oatmeal Cereal & Bananas *(Beech-Nut)*				4
Oatmeal Cereal with Applesauce & Bananas *(Beech-Nut)*				4
Papaya Tropical Fruit Dessert *(Beech-Nut)*			3	
Peaches & Yogurt *(Beech-Nut)*			3	
Pears & Applesauce *(Beech-Nut)*	★			
Pears & Pineapple *(Beech-Nut)*	★			
Peas & Carrots *(Beech-Nut)*	★			
Plums with Rice *(Beech-Nut)*			3	
Prunes with Pears *(Beech-Nut)*	★			
Rice Cereal with Applesauce & Bananas *(Beech-Nut)*			3	4

1 = High Fat	2 = High Sodium	3 = High Refined Sugar	5 = Cholesterol
1+ = Very High Fat	2+ = Very High Sodium	4 = Highly Processed	★= Better Choice

VARIETY *(Brand)* — RATING CODE

VARIETY *(Brand)*				
Turkey Dinner Supreme *(Beech-Nut)*		1		
Turkey Rice Dinner with Vegetables *(Beech-Nut)*	★			
Vanilla Custard Pudding *(Beech-Nut)*			3	
Vegetable Beef Dinner *(Beech-Nut)*		1		
Vegetable Chicken Dinner *(Beech-Nut)*	★			
Vegetable Ham Dinner *(Beech-Nut)*		1		
Vegetable Lamb Dinner *(Beech-Nut)*		1		
STAGE 3				
Applesauce *(Beech-Nut)*	★			
Applesauce & Bananas *(Beech-Nut)*	★			
Applesauce & Cherries *(Beech-Nut)*	★			
Apricots with Pears & Apples *(Beech-Nut)*	★			
Bananas with Pears & Apples *(Beech-Nut)*	★			
Beef & Egg Noodle Dinner *(Beech-Nut)*		1		
Carrots *(Beech-Nut)*			2	
Chicken Noodle Dinner *(Beech-Nut)*	★			
Cottage Cheese with Pineapple *(Beech-Nut)*				3
Fruit Dessert *(Beech-Nut)*	★			
Green Beans *(Beech-Nut)*	★			
Macaroni & Beef Dinner *(Beech-Nut)*		1		
Mixed Fruit & Yogurt *(Beech-Nut)*				3
Peaches *(Beech-Nut)*	★			
Pears *(Beech-Nut)*	★			
Spaghetti & Beef Dinner *(Beech-Nut)*		1		4
Sweet Potatoes *(Beech-Nut)*	★			
Table Time, Beef Stew *(Beech-Nut)*		1	2	
Table Time, Spaghetti Rings In Meat Sauce *(Beech-Nut)*			2	3 4
Table Time, Turkey Stew *(Beech-Nut)*		1	2	
Table Time, Vegetable Stew With Chicken *(Beech-Nut)*		1	2	
Table Time, Hearty Chicken With Stars Soup *(Beech-Nut)*		1	2	4
Turkey Rice Dinner *(Beech-Nut)*	★			
Vanilla Custard Pudding *(Beech-Nut)*				3

1 = High Fat   2 = High Sodium   3 = High Refined Sugar   5 = Cholesterol
1+ = Very High Fat   2+ = Very High Sodium   4 = Highly Processed   ★= Better Choice

VARIETY *(Brand)*   RATING CODE

Vegetable Beef Dinner *(Beech-Nut)*	1
Vegetable Chicken Dinner *(Beech-Nut)*	1

JUICES

Apple *(Beech-Nut)*	★
Apple Cherry *(Beech-Nut)*	★
Apple Cranberry *(Beech-Nut)*	★
Apple Grape *(Beech-Nut)*	★
Juice Plus *(Beech-Nut)*	★
Mixed Fruit *(Beech-Nut)*	★
Orange *(Beech-Nut)*	★
Pear *(Beech-Nut)*	★
Tropical Blend *(Beech-Nut)*	★
White Grape *(Beech-Nut)*	★

GERBER
FIRST FOODS

Applesauce *(Gerber)*	★	
Bananas *(Gerber)*	★	
Carrots *(Gerber)*	★	
Cereal, Barley *(Gerber)*		4
Cereal, High Protein *(Gerber)*		4
Cereal, Mixed *(Gerber)*		4
Cereal, Mixed with Bananas *(Gerber)*	3	4
Cereal, Oatmeal *(Gerber)*		4
Cereal, Oatmeal with Bananas *(Gerber)*	3	4
Cereal, Rice *(Gerber)*		4
Cereal, Rice with Bananas *(Gerber)*	3	4
Green Beans *(Gerber)*	★	
Peaches *(Gerber)*	★	
Pears *(Gerber)*	★	
Peas *(Gerber)*	★	

---

1 = High Fat	2 = High Sodium	3 = High Refined Sugar	5 = Cholesterol
1+ = Very High Fat	2+ = Very High Sodium	4 = Highly Processed	★= Better Choice

VARIETY *(Brand)*   RATING CODE

Variety (Brand)	★	1	2	3	4	5
Prunes *(Gerber)*	★					
Squash *(Gerber)*	★					
Sweet Potatoes *(Gerber)*	★					
STRAINED						
Apple Blueberry *(Gerber)*	★					
Applesauce *(Gerber)*	★					
Applesauce Apricot *(Gerber)*	★					
Apricots with Tapioca *(Gerber)*				3		
Banana Apple Dessert *(Gerber)*				3		
Bananas with Pineapple & Tapioca *(Gerber)*	★					
Bananas with Tapioca *(Gerber)*				3		
Beef *(Gerber)*		1				5
Beef Egg Noodle Dinner *(Gerber)*	★					
Beef with Vegetables Lean Meat Dinner *(Gerber)*	★					
Beets *(Gerber)*	★					
Carrots *(Gerber)*	★					
Cherry Vanilla Pudding *(Gerber)*				3		
Chicken *(Gerber)*		1+				5
Chicken Noodle Dinner *(Gerber)*					4	
Chicken with Vegetables Lean Meat Dinner *(Gerber)*	★					
Creamed Corn *(Gerber)*	★					
Dutch Apple Dessert *(Gerber)*					0	
Egg Yolks *(Gerber)*		1+				5
Fruit Dessert *(Gerber)*				3		
Garden Vegetables *(Gerber)*	★					
Green Beans *(Gerber)*	★					
Guava *(Gerber)*				3		
Ham *(Gerber)*		1				
Ham with Vegetables Lean Meat Dinner *(Gerber)*		1				
Hawaiian Delight *(Gerber)*				3		
Lamb *(Gerber)*		1				5
Macaroni Cheese Dinner *(Gerber)*					4	
Macaroni Tomato Beef Dinner *(Gerber)*					4	
Mango *(Gerber)*				3		

1 = High Fat   2 = High Sodium   3 = High Refined Sugar   5 = Cholesterol
1+ = Very High Fat   2+ = Very High Sodium   4 = Highly Processed   ★= Better Choice

VARIETY *(Brand)*   RATING CODE

Item	Rating
Mango, Bananas & Passion Fruit Juice *(Gerber)*	3
Mixed Cereal with Applesauce & Bananas *(Gerber)*	3 4
Mixed Vegetables *(Gerber)*	★
Oatmeal with Applesauce & Bananas *(Gerber)*	3 4
Papaya *(Gerber)*	3
Peach Cobbler *(Gerber)*	3
Peaches *(Gerber)*	3
Peaches Mango *(Gerber)*	3
Pear Pineapple *(Gerber)*	★
Pears *(Gerber)*	★
Peas *(Gerber)*	★
Plums with Tapioca *(Gerber)*	3
Prunes with Tapioca *(Gerber)*	★
Rice Cereal with Applesauce & Bananas *(Gerber)*	3 4
Spinach, Creamed *(Gerber)*	★
Squash *(Gerber)*	★
Sweet Potatoes *(Gerber)*	★
Tropical Fruits *(Gerber)*	3
Turkey *(Gerber)*	1+ 5
Turkey Rice Dinner *(Gerber)*	1
Turkey with Vegetables Lean Meat Dinner *(Gerber)*	1
Vanilla Custard Pudding *(Gerber)*	3
Veal *(Gerber)*	1
Vegetable Beef Dinner *(Gerber)*	1
Vegetable Chicken Dinner *(Gerber)*	★
Vegetable Ham Dinner *(Gerber)*	1
Vegetable Turkey Dinner *(Gerber)*	★

JUNIOR

Item	Rating
Apple Blueberry *(Gerber)*	★
Applesauce *(Gerber)*	★
Apricots with Tapioca *(Gerber)*	3
Bananas with Pineapple & Tapioca *(Gerber)*	★
Bananas with Tapioca *(Gerber)*	3
Beef *(Gerber)*	1

1 = High Fat   1+ = Very High Fat   2 = High Sodium   2+ = Very High Sodium   3 = High Refined Sugar   4 = Highly Processed   5 = Cholesterol   ★= Better Choice

BABY FOODS 97

VARIETY *(Brand)*   RATING CODE

Item (Brand)	★	1 / 1+	2 / 2+	3	4	5
Beef Egg Noodle Dinner *(Gerber)*					4	
Beef with Vegetables Lean Meat Dinner *(Gerber)*	★					
Biter Biscuits *(Gerber)*				3	4	
Broccoli, Carrots, Cheese *(Gerber)*	★					
Carrots *(Gerber)*	★					
Chicken *(Gerber)*		1+				5
Chicken Noodle Dinner *(Gerber)*					4	
Chicken Sticks *(Gerber)*		1+	2	3		5
Chicken with Vegetables Lean Meat Dinner *(Gerber)*	★					
Cookies, Animal Shapes *(Gerber)*				3	4	
Cookies, Arrowroot *(Gerber)*				3	4	
Dutch Apple Dessert *(Gerber)*				3		
Fruit Dessert *(Gerber)*				3		
Green Beans, Creamed *(Gerber)*	★					
Ham *(Gerber)*		1				5
Ham with Vegetables Lean Meat Dinner *(Gerber)*		1				
Hawaiian Delight *(Gerber)*				3		
Home Style Noodles & Beef, Chunky *(Gerber)*		1	2		4	
Macaroni Alphabets with Beef & Tomato Sauce *(Gerber)*			2	3	4	
Macaroni Tomato Beef Dinner *(Gerber)*					4	
Meat Sticks *(Gerber)*		1+	2+	3		5
Mixed Vegetables *(Gerber)*	★					
Mixed Cereal with Applesauce & Bananas *(Gerber)*				3		
Noodles & Chicken with Carrots & Peas, Chunky *(Gerber)*			2+		4	
Oatmeal with Applesauce & Bananas *(Gerber)*				3		
Peach Cobbler *(Gerber)*				3		
Peaches *(Gerber)*				3		
Pear Pineapple *(Gerber)*	★					
Pears *(Gerber)*	★					
Peas *(Gerber)*	★					
Plums with Tapioca *(Gerber)*				3		
Pretzels *(Gerber)*			2	3	4	
Rice Cereal with Mixed Fruit *(Gerber)*				3		

1 = High Fat   2 = High Sodium   3 = High Refined Sugar   5 = Cholesterol
1+ = Very High Fat   2+ = Very High Sodium   4 = Highly Processed   ★= Better Choice

VARIETY *(Brand)*   RATING CODE

Item	★	1 / 1+	2 / 2+	3	4	5
Rice with Beef & Tomato Sauce, Chunky *(Gerber)*			2	3	4	
Saucy Rice with Chicken, Chunky *(Gerber)*			2+		4	
Spaghetti, Tomato Sauce & Beef, Chunky *(Gerber)*			2	3	4	
Spaghetti, Tomato Sauce & Beef Dinner *(Gerber)*					4	
Squash *(Gerber)*	★					
Sweet Potatoes *(Gerber)*	★					
Turkey *(Gerber)*		1+				5
Turkey Rice Dinner *(Gerber)*					4	
Turkey Sticks *(Gerber)*		1+	2	3		5
Turkey with Vegetables Lean Meat Dinner *(Gerber)*		1				
Vanilla Custard Pudding *(Gerber)*				3		
Veal *(Gerber)*		1				
Vegetable Beef Dinner *(Gerber)*	★					
Vegetable Chicken Dinner *(Gerber)*	★					
Vegetable Ham Dinner *(Gerber)*	★					
Vegetable Turkey Dinner *(Gerber)*	★					
Vegetables & Beef, Chunky *(Gerber)*		1	2+			
Vegetables & Chicken, Chunky *(Gerber)*		1	2+			
Vegetables & Ham, Chunky *(Gerber)*		1	2			
Vegetables & Turkey, Chunky *(Gerber)*			2+			
JUICES						
Apple *(Gerber)*	★					
Apple Banana *(Gerber)*	★					
Apple Cherry *(Gerber)*	★					
Apple Grape *(Gerber)*	★					
Apple Peach *(Gerber)*	★					
Apple Plum *(Gerber)*	★					
Apple Prune *(Gerber)*	★					
Grape *(Gerber)*	★					
Mixed Fruit *(Gerber)*	★					
Orange *(Gerber)*	★					
Pear *(Gerber)*	★					
White Grape *(Gerber)*	★					

1 = High Fat	2 = High Sodium	3 = High Refined Sugar 5 = Cholesterol
1+ = Very High Fat	2+ = Very High Sodium	4 = Highly Processed ★= Better Choice

VARIETY (Brand)   RATING CODE

	★	1 / 1+	2	3	4	5
HEINZ						
BEGINNER						
Applesauce *(Heinz)*	★					
Bananas *(Heinz)*	★					
Carrots *(Heinz)*	★					
Cereal, Hi-Protein *(Heinz)*					4	
Cereal, Mixed *(Heinz)*					4	
Cereal, Oatmeal *(Heinz)*					4	
Green Beans *(Heinz)*	★					
Peaches *(Heinz)*	★					
Pears *(Heinz)*	★					
Peas *(Heinz)*	★					
Squash *(Heinz)*	★					
Sweet Potatoes *(Heinz)*	★					
STRAINED						
Apples & Apricots *(Heinz)*	★					
Apples & Cranberries with Tapioca *(Heinz)*				3		
Apples & Pears *(Heinz)*	★					
Applesauce *(Heinz)*	★					
Apricot Yogurt *(Heinz)*				3		
Apricots with Tapioca *(Heinz)*				3		
Banana Pudding *(Heinz)*				3		
Banana Yogurt *(Heinz)*				3		
Bananas & Pineapple with Tapioca *(Heinz)*				3		
Bananas with Tapioca *(Heinz)*				3		
Beef & Beef Broth *(Heinz)*		1+				5
Beef & Egg Noodles *(Heinz)*					4	
Beets *(Heinz)*	★					
Blueberry Yogurt *(Heinz)*				3		
Carrots *(Heinz)*			2			
Chicken & Chicken Broth *(Heinz)*		1+				5
Chicken Noodle Dinner *(Heinz)*					4	
Chicken Soup *(Heinz)*	★					

1 = High Fat   2 = High Sodium   3 = High Refined Sugar   5 = Cholesterol
1+ = Very High Fat   2+ = Very High Sodium   4 = Highly Processed   ★= Better Choice

VARIETY *(Brand)*   RATING CODE

Creamed Corn *(Heinz)*			3	
Creamed Peas *(Heinz)*	★			
Custard Pudding *(Heinz)*			3	
Dutch Apple Dessert *(Heinz)*			3	
Fruit Dessert *(Heinz)*			3	
Green Beans *(Heinz)*	★			
Lamb & Lamb Broth *(Heinz)*	1+			5
Liver & Liver Broth *(Heinz)*	1			5
Macaroni, Tomatoes & Beef *(Heinz)*			4	
Mixed Cereal with Apples & Bananas *(Heinz)*			3	
Mixed Fruit Yogurt *(Heinz)*			3	
Mixed Vegetables *(Heinz)*	★			
Oatmeal with Apples & Bananas *(Heinz)*			3	
Peach Cobbler *(Heinz)*			3	
Peach Yogurt *(Heinz)*			3	
Peaches *(Heinz)*			3	
Pear Yogurt *(Heinz)*			3	
Pears *(Heinz)*	★			
Pears & Pineapple *(Heinz)*	★			
Pineapple Orange *(Heinz)*			3	
Plums with Tapioca *(Heinz)*			3	
Prunes with Tapioca *(Heinz)*			3	
Rice Cereal with Apples & Bananas *(Heinz)*			3	
Squash *(Heinz)*	★			
Strawberry Banana Yogurt *(Heinz)*			3	
Strawberry Yogurt *(Heinz)*			3	
Sweet Potatoes *(Heinz)*	★			
Turkey & Turkey Broth *(Heinz)*	1+			5
Turkey Rice Dinner with Vegetables *(Heinz)*	★			
Tutti Frutti *(Heinz)*			3	
Veal & Veal Broth *(Heinz)*	1			
Vegetables & Bacon *(Heinz)*	1			
Vegetables & Beef *(Heinz)*	★			

1 = High Fat	2 = High Sodium	3 = High Refined Sugar	5 = Cholesterol
1+ = Very High Fat	2+ = Very High Sodium	4 = Highly Processed	★ = Better Choice

VARIETY (Brand)   RATING CODE

	★	1 / 1+ / 2	3	4	5
Vegetables & Ham (Heinz)	★				
Vegetables & Lamb (Heinz)	★				
Vegetables, Egg Noodles & Chicken (Heinz)				4	
Vegetables, Egg Noodles & Turkey (Heinz)				4	
JUNIOR					
Apples & Apricots (Heinz)	★				
Apples & Cranberries with Tapioca (Heinz)			3		
Apples & Pears (Heinz)	★				
Applesauce (Heinz)	★				
Apricots with Tapioca (Heinz)			3		
Bananas & Pineapple with Tapioca (Heinz)			3		
Bananas with Tapioca (Heinz)			3		
Beef & Beef Broth (Heinz)		1+			5
Carrots (Heinz)		2			
Chicken & Chicken Broth (Heinz)		1			5
Chicken Noodle Dinner (Heinz)				4	
Creamed Corn (Heinz)			3		
Custard Pudding (Heinz)			3		
Dutch Apple (Heinz)			3		
Egg Noodles & Beef (Heinz)				4	
Fruit Dessert (Heinz)			3		
Macaroni, Tomatoes & Beef (Heinz)				4	
Peaches (Heinz)			3		
Pears (Heinz)	★				
Pineapple Orange (Heinz)			3		
Spaghetti, Tomato Sauce & Meat (Heinz)				4	
Sweet Potatoes (Heinz)	★				
Turkey Rice Dinner with Vegetables (Heinz)				4	
Tutti Frutti (Heinz)			3		
Vegetables & Beef (Heinz)	★				
Vegetables, Egg Noodles & Chicken (Heinz)				4	
Vegetables, Egg Noodles & Turkey (Heinz)		1		4	

1 = High Fat   2 = High Sodium   3 = High Refined Sugar   5 = Cholesterol
1+ = Very High Fat   2+ = Very High Sodium   4 = Highly Processed   ★ = Better Choice

VARIETY (Brand)	RATING CODE
JUICES	
Apple *(Heinz)*	★
Apple Apricot *(Heinz)*	★
Apple Banana *(Heinz)*	★
Apple Cherry *(Heinz)*	★
Apple Cranberry *(Heinz)*	★
Apple Grape *(Heinz)*	★
Apple Peach *(Heinz)*	★
Apple Pineapple *(Heinz)*	★
Apple Prune *(Heinz)*	★
Mixed Fruit *(Heinz)*	★
Orange *(Heinz)*	★
Orange Apple *(Heinz)*	★
Orange Apple Banana *(Heinz)*	★
Pear *(Heinz)*	★

BAKING ITEMS

Baking ingredients, such as flour and corn meal, are always the best choice when the whole grain is used. There are many good flours on the market: wheat, rice, rye, amaranth, soy, and so on. By far the best choices are those which are made from the whole grain. Refined flour such as bleached or unbleached wheat flour has had many vitamins and minerals removed as well as most of its fiber.

As for corn meal, most varieties on our shelves have been degerminated. Obviously, this means that we have been robbed of the corn germ nutrients. Generally, manufacturers remove the germ in order for corn meal to have a longer shelf life. It won't attract bugs or become rancid as quickly when it has been degerminated.

Since whole grains are not highly processed, they attract bugs. Bugs know a good thing when they see it! If you don't use these products quickly, store them in the refrigerator or freezer. This is where I put mine.

As for baking powder, I want to avoid the aluminum that is in most brands of baking powder such as *Calumet* and *Clabber Girl*. Personally, I use the *Rumford* brand. Of course, baking powder with aluminum is not included in *The Food Bible*.

VARIETY *(Brand)* RATING CODE

VARIETY (Brand)	★		
BAKING ITEMS			
CORN MEAL			
Blue Corn Meal *(Arrowhead Mills)*	★		
Hi-Lysine Corn Meal *(Arrowhead Mills)*	★		
White Corn Meal *(Alber's)*			4
White Corn Meal *(Aunt Jemima)*			4
White Corn Meal *(Hodgson Mill)*	★		
White Corn Meal *(Quaker)*			4
White Corn Meal *(Shawnee's)*			4
White Cream Corn Meal *(Dixie Lily)*			4
White Water-Ground Corn Meal *(Dixie Lily)*			4
Yellow Corn Meal *(Alber's)*			4
Yellow Corn Meal *(Arrowhead Mills)*	★		
Yellow Corn Meal *(Aunt Jemima)*			4
Yellow Corn Meal *(Dixie Lily)*			4
Yellow Corn Meal *(Hodgson Mill)*	★		
Yellow Corn Meal *(Martha White)*			4
Yellow Corn Meal *(Mrs. Wright's)*			4
Yellow Corn Meal *(Quaker)*			4
Yellow Corn Meal *(Shawnee's)*			4
Yellow Corn Meal *(Stone-Buhr)*	★		
FLOUR			
All Purpose, Bleached *(Gold Medal)*			4
All Purpose, Bleached *(Gladiola)*			4
All Purpose, Bleached *(Martha White)*			4
All Purpose, Bleached *(Mrs. Wright's)*			4
All Purpose, Bleached *(Pillsbury)*			4
All Purpose, Bleached *(Rainbow)*			4
Amaranth *(Arrowhead Mills)*	★		
Barley *(Arrowhead Mills)*	★		
Brown Rice *(Arrowhead Mills)*	★		
Buckwheat *(Arrowhead Mills)*	★		
Buckwheat *(Hodgson Mill)*	★		
Dark Rye *(Stone-Buhr)*	★		

1 = High Fat   2 = High Sodium   3 = High Refined Sugar   5 = Cholesterol
1+ = Very High Fat   2+ = Very High Sodium   4 = Highly Processed   ★= Better Choice

VARIETY *(Brand)*   RATING CODE

VARIETY (Brand)	★			4
Ezekiel *(Arrowhead Mills)*	★			
Garbanzo *(Arrowhead Mills)*	★			
Graham *(Hodgson Mill)*	★			
Graham *(Stone-Buhr)*	★			
Millet *(Arrowhead Mills)*	★			
Oat *(Arrowhead Mills)*	★			
Pastry *(Arrowhead Mills)*	★			
Quinoa *(Ancient Harvest)*	★			
Rye Flour *(Arrowhead Mills)*	★			
Rye Flour *(Elam's)*	★			
Rye Flour *(Hodgson Mill)*	★			
Sauce 'n Gravy Flour *(Gold Medal)*				4
Semolina *(Stone-Buhr)*				4
Softasilk *(Betty Crocker)*				4
Soy *(Arrowhead Mills)*	★			
Soy *(Stone-Buhr)*	★			
Teff *(Arrowhead Mills)*	★			
Triticale *(Arrowhead Mills)*	★			
Two Cup, Bleached *(Martha White)*				4
Unbleached *(Arrowhead Mills)*				4
Unbleached *(Gold Medal)*				4
Unbleached *(Hodgson Mill)*				4
Unbleached *(Mrs. Wright's)*				4
Unbleached *(Stone-Buhr)*				4
Whole Wheat *(Arrowhead Mills)*	★			
Whole Wheat *(Elam's)*	★			
Whole Wheat *(Gold Medal)*	★			
Whole Wheat *(Hodgson Mill)*	★			
Whole Wheat *(Pillsbury)*	★			
Whole Wheat *(Stone-Buhr)*	★			
Whole Wheat Pastry *(Stone-Buhr)*	★			
Wondra *(Gold Medal)*				4

1 = High Fat	2 = High Sodium	3 = High Refined Sugar	5 = Cholesterol
1+ = Very High Fat	2+ = Very High Sodium	4 = Highly Processed	★= Better Choice

BAKING MIXES

I like the convenience of mixes just like the next person, so I keep them in my pantry. Many baking mixes did not make *The Food Bible* because of aluminum in the baking powder. Some also contain cottonseed oil. As an example:

Betty Crocker Bisquick	cottonseed oil & aluminum
Duncan Hines Fudge Cake Mix	aluminum, artificial flavor & artificial color

The best choice mixes feature whole grains. Obviously, these contain more nutrients, fiber and flavor than their highly processed cousins.

VARIETY *(Brand)*   RATING CODE

VARIETY (Brand)	★	2+ / 2	4
BAKING MIXES			
Baking Mix, Whole Wheat *(Hain)*		2+	
Baking Mix, Whole Wheat Insta-Bake *(Hodgson Mill)*		2	
Biscuit & Pancake Mix, Buttermilk *(Health Valley)*		2	
Biscuit Mix *(Arrowhead Mills)*		2	
Biscuit Mix, Buttermilk *(Hodgson Mill)*		2	
Corn Bread & Muffin Mix, Whole Grain *(Hodgson Mill)*	★		
Corn Bread Mix *(Arrowhead Mills)*		2	
Corn Bread Mix, Jalapeño *(Hodgson Mill)*	★		
Corn Meal Mix, Self-Rising *(Martha White)*		2+	4
Corn Meal Mix, Self-Rising Buttermilk *(Aunt Jemima)*		2+	4
Corn Meal Mix, Self-Rising White *(Aunt Jemima)*		2+	4
Corn Meal Mix, Self-Rising White *(Dixie Lily)*		2+	4
Corn Meal Mix, Self-Rising White *(Hodgson Mill)*		2+	
Corn Meal Mix, Self-Rising Yellow *(Aunt Jemima)*		2+	4
Corn Meal Mix, Self-Rising Yellow *(Hodgson Mill)*		2+	
Gingerbread Mix, Whole Wheat *(Hodgson Mill)*	★		
Muffin Mix, Apple-Spice Oat Bran *(Arrowhead Mills)*		2	
Muffin Mix, Apple Cinnamon Oat Bran *(Hain)*		2+	
Muffin Mix, Banana Nut Oat Bran *(Hain)*		2+	
Muffin Mix, Blue Corn *(Arrowhead Mills)*		2	
Muffin Mix, Bran *(Arrowhead Mills)*	★		
Muffin Mix, Bran *(Hodgson Mill)*		2	
Muffin Mix, Raspberry Spice Oat Bran *(Hain)*		2+	
Muffin Mix, Wheat-Free Oat Bran *(Arrowhead Mills)*		2	
Muffin Mix, Whole Wheat *(Hodgson Mill)*	★		
Tortilla Mix, Corn *(Quaker)*			4
OTHER			
Baking Powder *(Rumford)*		2+	
Baking Soda *(Arm & Hammer)*		2+	
Corn Starch *(Argo)*	★		
Corn Starch *(Cream)*	★		

1 = High Fat	2 = High Sodium	3 = High Refined Sugar	5 = Cholesterol
1+ = Very High Fat	2+ = Very High Sodium	4 = Highly Processed	★= Better Choice

BEANS (LEGUMES)

These kinds of beans are wonderful. They're excellent energy foods, an excellent source of complex carbohydrates and fiber, and they're "brim full" of nutrients.

The canned varieties are easy to keep on hand and pull out when we want them. You'll notice that a lot of brands are not in *The Food Bible*, and this is because of the additive EDTA, and in some cases, cottonseed oil. For example: *Green Giant* Kidney Beans contains EDTA, and *Ranch Style* Beans contains cottonseed oil. Also, most canned refried beans contain lard, a highly saturated fat.

All brands of plain, dried beans that I have seen are excellent foods without additives and preservatives.

Personally, I'm a bean lover, so I keep my shelves well stocked. Since there is quite a difference in price, I will choose the best buy. I also like the convenience of the dried bean flakes. They're great to take when traveling — just add hot water, and they're ready to eat. I've become particularly fond of Instant Beans by *Fantastic Foods* and Bean Flakes by *Taste Adventure*.

VARIETY *(Brand)*   RATING CODE

BEANS (LEGUMES)	
BOXED	
Black Bean Flakes *(Taste Adventure)*	2+
Black Beans, Instant *(Fantastic Foods)*	2+
Pinto Bean Flakes *(Taste Adventure)*	2+
Refried Beans, Instant *(Fantastic Foods)*	2+
CANNED	
Baked Beans *(B & M)*	2+ 3
Baked Beans *(Whole Earth)*	2+
Baked Beans, Boston *(Health Valley)*	3
Baked Beans, Boston - No Salt *(Health Valley)*	3
Baked Beans, Brick Oven *(S & W)*	2+ 3
Baked Beans, Maple Sugar *(S & W)*	2+ 3
Beans, Micro Cup *(Ranch Style)*	2+
Black Beans *(Goya)*	2+
Black Beans *(La Preferida)*	2+
Black Beans *(Progresso)*	2+
Butter Beans *(Bush's)*	2+
Butter Beans, Speckled *(Bush's)*	2+
Cajun Beans *(S & W)*	2+
Chili Beans *(Ashley's)*	2+
Chili Beans *(Casa Fiesta)*	2+
Chili Beans *(Ellis)*	2+
Chili Beans *(Town House)*	2+
Chili Beans in Sauce *(Chili Man)*	2+
Chili Beans in Sauce, Jalapeño Style *(Chili Man)*	2+
Crowder Peas *(Griffin's)*	2+
Fava Beans *(Progresso)*	2+
Field Peas & Snaps *(Griffin's)*	2+
Garbanzo Beans *(Casa Fiesta)*	2+
Garbanzo Beans *(Flora)*	2+
Garden Salad Beans *(Read)*	2+ 3
Great Northern Beans *(Bush's)*	2+
Great Northern Beans *(Eden)*	2+

VARIETY *(Brand)*   RATING CODE

VARIETY (Brand)	RATING CODE
Great Northern Beans *(Hanover)*	2+
Great Northern Beans *(Randall)*	2+
Great Northern Beans *(Sun-Vista)*	2+
Kidney Beans *(S & W)*	2+
Kidney Beans, Lite *(S & W)*	2
Maple Sugar Beans *(S & W)*	2+ 3
Mexican Style Beans *(Allen's)*	2+
Mexican Style Beans *(Griffins)*	2+
Mexican Style Beans *(Rainbow)*	2+
Pinto Beans *(Casa Fiesta)*	2+
Pinto Beans *(Eden)*	2+
Pinto Beans *(Randall)*	2+
Pork & Beans *(Campbell's)*	2+
Pork & Beans *(Rainbow)*	2+
Pork & Beans *(Town House)*	2+
Pork & Beans Showboat *(Bush's)*	2+
Pork & Beans, Wagon Master *(Allen's)*	2+ 3
Red Beans *(Bush's)*	2+
Refried Beans *(Little Bear)*	2
Refried Beans *(Zapata)*	2+
Refried Beans, Spicy *(Little Bear)*	2
Refried Beans, Spicy *(Zapata)*	2+
Refried Beans, Vegetarian *(Old El Paso)*	2+
Roman Beans *(Goya)*	2+
Three Bean Salad *(Read)*	2+ 3
Vegetarian Beans *(Heinz)*	2+
Vegetarian Beans with Miso *(Health Valley)*	2
White Beans in Tomato Sauce *(Rena)*	2+
DRY	
Bean Soup Mix *(Ozark Beans)*	★
Bean Soup Mix, Grandma's Special *(Ozark Beans)*	★
Bean Soup Mix, Split Pea & Bean *(Ozark Beans)*	★

1 = High Fat   2 = High Sodium   3 = High Refined Sugar   5 = Cholesterol
1+ = Very High Fat   2+ = Very High Sodium   4 = Highly Processed   ★= Better Choice

VARIETY *(Brand)*   RATING CODE

Variety (Brand)	Rating Code
Dry Beans *(Adobe Milling)*	★
Dry Beans *(Benco)*	★
Dry Beans *(Evans)*	★
Dry Beans *(Goya)*	★
Dry Beans *(Ham Beens)*	★
Dry Beans *(Hodgson Mill)*	★
Dry Beans *(Hurst's)*	★
Dry Beans *(Iberia)*	★
Dry Beans *(La Cina)*	★
Dry Beans *(La Preferida)*	★
Dry Beans *(Martha White)*	★
Dry Beans *(Tender Cook)*	★
Dry Beans *(Town House)*	★

BEVERAGES AND
SPORT DRINKS

This is a very unusual group in that it covers many categories of drinks, and each product within a category can vary a tremendous amount.

I have chosen not to list mineral waters, spring waters, sparkling waters, etc. because the sodium content can vary from very high to almost non-existent, and many times the sodium information is not available. This variance depends on the source of the water as well as what the bottler adds or doesn't add.

Notice that I have included some soda pop, but not the diet varieties. They contain a wide assortment of additives and preservatives, including aspartame (NutraSweet), saccharin, sodium benzoate, BHA, artificial color and artificial flavor. Most of the hot cocoa mixes contain the tropical oils — coconut oil, palm oil or palm kernel oil.

NOTE: I feel that we should not drink any beverage from an aluminum can. This includes soft drinks, juice, beer and so on. Fortunately, we have a choice. We can drink these beverages from bottles.

There are some very good beverage choices in this group. I especially like the soy drinks by *Westbrae Natural*. The cocoa-flavored Westsoy Lite is my favorite. The sport drinks by *R. W. Knudsen* are excellent choices with no refined sugar. Sport drinks usually contain refined sugar as well as additives and preservatives, such as *10-K* which contains sodium benzoate, potassium sorbate and artificial color.

Choose wisely from this group, and you can get some top-notch drinks.

VARIETY *(Brand)* — RATING CODE

VARIETY (Brand)	★	1	1+	2	3	4
BEVERAGES AND SPORT DRINKS						
BEVERAGES						
Black Cherry Soda *(Natur`ale 90)*						4
Bloody Mary Mix *(Tabasco)*				2		4
Carob Malted Mix *(Caroba)*					3	
Carob Mix *(Caroba)*					3	
Carob Mix *(Chatfield's)*					3	
Coffee Substitute, Cafix *(Cafix)*	★					
Coke, Caffeine Free *(Coca Cola)*					3	4
Cola, Caffeine Free *(Natur`ale 90)*						4
Cola, Natural Soda *(Corr)*						4
Cream Soda *(Natur`ale 90)*						4
Daiquiri Mix, Boxed *(Holland House)*					3	4
Ginger Beer *(Natur`ale 90)*						4
Ginseng Rush *(American Ginseng)*						4
Juice Squeeze, Mountain Raspberry *(Crystal Geyser)*	★					
Juice Squeeze, Orange & Passion Fruit *(Crystal Geyser)*	★					
Juice Squeeze, Passion Fruit & Mango *(Crystal Geyser)*	★					
Juice Squeeze, Pink Lemonade *(Crystal Geyser)*	★					
Juice Squeeze, Wild Berry *(Crystal Geyser)*	★					
Lemon-Lime Soda *(Natur`ale 90)*						4
Orange Soda *(Natur`ale 90)*						4
Pepsi, Caffeine Free *(Pepsi Cola)*					3	4
Punch Soda, Natural Fruit *(Natur`ale 90)*						4
Raspberry Soda *(Natur`ale 90)*						4
7-Up *(7-Up)*					3	4
Soy *(West Soy)*		1			3	
Soy Creamer, Powdered *(Solait)*			1+		3	
Soy Moo *(Health Valley)*		1			3	
Soy, American Original *(Ah Soy)*		1			3	
Soy, Carob *(Ah Soy)*					3	
Soy, Carob *(Edensoy)*					3	
Soy, Carob Malted *(Westbrae Natural)*		1			3	
Soy, Carob Supreme *(Vitasoy)*					3	
Soy, Cocoa Mint-Malted *(Westbrae Natural)*		1			3	

1 = High Fat   2 = High Sodium   3 = High Refined Sugar   5 = Cholesterol
1+ = Very High Fat   2+ = Very High Sodium   4 = Highly Processed   ★= Better Choice

VARIETY *(Brand)*   RATING CODE

	1	3	
Soy, Creamy Original *(Vitasoy)*	1	3	
Soy, Dutch Cocoa *(Ah Soy)*	1	3	
Soy, Edensoy Original *(Eden Foods)*		3	
Soy, Edensoy Vanilla *(Eden Foods)*		3	
Soy, Original *(Ah Soy)*	1	3	
Soy, Powdered *(Solait)*	1	3	
Soy, Vanilla Delite *(Vitasoy)*		3	
Soy, Vanilla Malted *(Westbrae Natural)*	1	3	
Tom Collins Mix, Boxed *(Holland House)*		3	
Westsoy Lite, Cocoa *(Westbrae Natural)*	★		
Westsoy Lite, Plain *(Westbrae Natural)*	★		
Westsoy Lite, Vanilla *(Westbrae Natural)*	★		
SPORT DRINKS			
Berry Punch *(Power Burst)*		3	
Citrus *(Freestyle)*		3	
Lemon Lime *(Freestyle)*		3	
Lemon Lime *(Power Burst)*		3	
Lemon Recharge *(R. W. Knudsen)*	★		
Lemonade *(Power Burst)*		3	
Orange Recharge *(R. W. Knudsen)*	★		
Sprint Sports Beverage *(After the Fall)*	★		
Tangerine *(Freestyle)*		3	
Tropical Recharge *(R. W. Knudsen)*	★		
Ultra Fuel, Fruit Punch *(Twinlab)*		3	
Ultra Fuel, Lemon Lime *(Twinlab)*		3	
Ultra Fuel, Orange *(Twinlab)*		3	

BREADS AND BREADSTUFFS

I am really disappointed in most of our bread choices on the market. We have the white breads that are so highly processed with additives and preservatives and even some whole grain types with additives and preservatives. For example: *Roman Meal* puts out a good-looking bread but with calcium propionate and potassium bromate added; so it didn't make *The Food Bible*. There are a few good ones, and if we keep asking for and buying the good ones, the manufacturers will eventually get the message, and we'll begin seeing more good choices. *Caution*: Just because a bread is dark in color and says "wheat bread," this does not mean that it is whole wheat bread. Manufacturers are good at coloring bread so it appears whole wheat. To be whole wheat bread, the very first ingredient must say *whole wheat flour*. The whole grain breads are an excellent food choice which I rate very high.

Since I eat quite a lot of bread, it is important for me to choose varieties that are whole grain. In other words, I want the most nutrients for my calories. As you can see, we are beginning to get some good choices.

VARIETY *(Brand)*

RATING CODE

BREADS AND BREADSTUFFS			
BREADS			
Bran for Life *(Food for Life)*		2	
Bran'nola, Country Oat *(Arnold)*		2	4
Bran'nola, Country Oat *(Brownberry)*		2	4
Bran'nola, Country Oat *(Oroweat)*		2	4
Bran'nola, Dark Wheat *(Arnold)*		2	
Bran'nola, Dark Wheat *(Oroweat)*		2	
Bran'nola, Nutty Grains *(Arnold)*			4
Bran'nola, Original *(Brownberry)*		2	4
Bran'nola, Original *(Oroweat)*		2	4
Bran'nola, Rice Bran *(Oroweat)*		2	4
Brown Bread, Raisin *(B & M)*		2 3	
Cinnamon Raisin *(Food for Life)*	★		
Cinnamon Raisin *(Rudi's)*	★		
Cracked Wheat *(Rudi's)*	★		
Dill Rye *(Brownberry)*		2	4
Honey Oat Berry *(Oroweat)*		2	
Honey Wheat Berry *(Arnold)*		2	
Honey Wheat Berry *(Oroweat)*		2	
Honey White *(Rudi's)*		2	4
Honey Whole Wheat *(Rudi's)*		2	
Jewish Light Rye *(Rudi's)*		2	4
Millet *(Food for Life)*	★		
Multigrain Oat *(Rudi's)*		2	
Oat Bran *(Shiloh Farms)*	★		
Oat Bran, No Sodium *(Shiloh Farms)*	★		
Oatberry, No Oil *(Alvarado St. Bakery)*	★		
Oatmeal *(Brownberry)*		2	4
Raisin *(Sun-Maid)*		2	4
Rice *(Food for Life)*		2	4
Rocky Mountain Sourdough *(Rudi's)*		2	
7 Grains, Sprouted *(Food for Life)*	★		
Sprouted 5 Grain *(Shiloh Farms)*	★		
Sprouted 10 Grain *(Shiloh Farms)*	★		

1 = High Fat	2 = High Sodium	3 = High Refined Sugar
1+ = Very High Fat	2+ = Very High Sodium	4 = Highly Processed

5 = Cholesterol	
★= Better Choice	

VARIETY *(Brand)*   RATING CODE

VARIETY (Brand)			
Sprouted Barley *(Alvarado St. Bakery)*	★		
Sprouted Grain, Ezekiel 4:9 *(Food for Life)*	★		
Sprouted Grain, Ezekiel 4:9 - Low Sodium *(Food for Life)*	★		
Sprouted Rye Seed *(Alvarado St. Bakery)*	★		
Sprouted Wheat *(Alvarado St. Bakery)*	★		
Sunflower Oat *(Rudi's)*	★		
Wheat Bran *(Brownberry)*		2	4
Wheat, Natural *(Brownberry)*		2	
Whole Wheat *(Pritikin)*	★		
Whole Wheat *(Shiloh Farms)*	★		
Whole Wheat, 100% *(Earth Grains)*		2	
BREADSTUFFS			
Bagels, Cinnamon Raisin *(Bagel Works)*		2	4
Bagels, Onion *(Bagel Works)*		2	4
Bagels, Onion Poppy Seed *(Alvarado St. Bakery)*	★		
Bagels, Onion Garlic *(Garden of Eatin')*	★		
Bagels, Plain *(Bagel Works)*		2	4
Bagels, Raisin *(Garden of Eatin')*	★		
Bagels, Sesame *(Garden of Eatin')*	★		
Bagels, Sprouted Wheat *(Alvarado St. Bakery)*	★		
Bagels, Swedish Rye *(Garden of Eatin')*	★		
Breadsticks, Garlic *(Angonoa's)*		2	4
Breadsticks, Italian *(Angonoa's)*		2	4
Breadsticks, Mini Whole Wheat *(Angonoa's)*		2	
Breadsticks, Onion *(Angonoa's)*		2	4
Breadsticks, Sesame Royale *(Angonoa's)*		2	4
Breadsticks, Sesame Whole Wheat *(Gadetto's)*		2	
Breadsticks, Whole Wheat Sesame *(Oroweat)*		2	
Croutons *(Jaclyn's)*		2	
Croutons, 'Toasted Only' *(Brownberry)*		2	4
Croutons, Plain *(Gourmet Award)*			4
Dressing, Corn Bread *(Oroweat)*		2	4
Dressing, Seasoned *(Oroweat)*		2+	4

VARIETY *(Brand)*   RATING CODE

English Muffins *(Pritikin)*	★		
Finger Rolls, Whole Wheat *(Food for Life)*	★		
Hamburger Buns *(Food for Life)*	★		
Hamburger Buns, Bran'nola *(Arnold)*		2		4
Hot Dog Buns, Whole Wheat *(Cybro's)*		2		
Ice Cream Cone Cups *(Disney)*			3	4
Ice Cream Cone Cups *(Keebler)*			3	4
Ice Cream Cones, Waffle *(Colosso-Cone)*			3	4
Ice Cream Cones, Waffle *(Disney)*			3	4
Ice Cream Cones, Whole Wheat *(Tree of Life)*			3	
Pita Bread, Swedish Rye *(Garden of Eatin')*	★			
Pita Bread, Whole Wheat *(Garden of Eatin')*	★			
Pita Puffs, Whole Wheat *(Garden of Eatin')*		2		
Pizza Crust, Whole Wheat *(Tree Tavern)*	★			
Rolls, Whole Wheat *(Matthews)*		2		
Stuffing Mix, Herb *(Brownberry)*		2+		4
Stuffing Mix, Sage & Onion *(Brownberry)*		2+		4

1 = High Fat	2 = High Sodium	3 = High Refined Sugar	5 = Cholesterol
1+ = Very High Fat	2+ = Very High Sodium	4 = Highly Processed	★= Better Choice

BUTTER AND MARGARINE

It is very difficult to find a margarine that doesn't contain additives and preservatives — EDTA, potassium sorbate, sodium benzoate, artificial flavor or artificial color. For example: *Weight Watchers* Margarine contains potassium sorbate and EDTA. In addition to the additives and preservatives, oils used to make margarines have to be hardened (hydrogenated) in order to make them firm enough to spread. To me, that's about like eating candle wax.

In my opinion, real butter is a better choice. Society seems to be hung up on the cholesterol in butter, but a single serving, one teaspoon, has only 11 mg. of cholesterol. That's not even enough cholesterol to be rated in *The Food Bible*. Now, don't get me wrong. I'm not promoting butter; I'm just saying that I feel that butter is a better choice than margarine.

Personally, I try to avoid most margarines because of the unhealthy ingredients. And, I limit my butter consumption. I would, however, like to share a recipe with you for a butter spread that I use and that I have recommended to all my clients. It has 5 ½ mg. of cholesterol per serving, no additives or preservatives, and is less saturated than margarine.

BUTTER SPREAD
1 pound butter, lightly salted
2 cups safflower oil
Mix in blender; pour into containers and refrigerate.

I think you'll like this spread. Just remember that it, as well as margarine or butter, is 100% fat. So use sparingly.

VARIETY *(Brand)*   RATING CODE

VARIETY (Brand)	RATING CODE
BUTTER AND MARGARINE	
BUTTER	
Butter *(Alta•Dena)*	1+
Butter *(Lucerne)*	1+
Butter *(Schepps)*	1+
Butter, No Salt *(Cabot)*	1+
Butter, No Salt *(Land-O-Lakes)*	1+
Butter, Salted *(Challenge)*	1+
Butter, Salted *(Tillamook)*	1+
Butter, Unsalted *(Challenge)*	1+
Butter, Unsalted *(Lucerne)*	1+
Butter, Unsalted *(Tillamook)*	1+
Butter, Whipped, Lightly Salted *(Challenge)*	1+
Butter, Whipped, Lightly Salted *(Land-O-Lakes)*	1+
Butter, Whipped, Salt Free *(Falfurrias)*	1+
Butter, Whipped, Unsalted *(Challenge)*	1+
Butter, Whipped, Unsalted *(Land-O-Lakes)*	1+
MARGARINE	
Margarine, Safflower *(Hain)*	1+ 2
Margarine, Soft Safflower *(Hain)*	1+ 2
Margarine, Soya *(Tree of Life)*	1+
Margarine, Soya, Salt Free *(Tree of Life)*	1+
Margarine, Soybean *(Old Stone Mill)*	1+
Margarine, Soybean, Salt Free *(Old Stone Mill)*	1+
Margarine, Unsalted Safflower *(Hain)*	1+

CEREALS

There are many excellent cereals available, and they provide an excellent way to start our day. Many cereals which appear healthful could be listed here if it weren't for the preservatives BHA, BHT and sulfites — among others. Notice that most of the kids' favorites are not listed either. The major reason here is the artificial colors and flavors that are used.

EXAMPLES:

Post Fruity Pebbles	artificial color, artificial flavor & BHA
General Mills Lucky Charms	artificial flavor & artificial color
Kellogg's Fruitful Bran	sulfur dioxide

Cereal companies are very competitive and manufacturers have created some "catchy" healthful-looking pictures and quotes. It's easy to go from very good to very bad when picking cereals; however, I rate this group of cereals listed here as very good and nutritious.

I definitely enjoy my cereal! I'll have a bowl most every morning and most times with wheat germ added. Many times I'll top some yogurt with a crunchy cereal. I use some cereals in pancakes, in casseroles and on top of casseroles. When we're talking quick and easy meals, a wise choice on the cereal aisle can be an easy way to boost vitamin, mineral and fiber intake.

VARIETY *(Brand)*   RATING CODE

Variety (Brand)	Rating Code
CEREALS	
All-Bran *(Kellogg's)*	2+
Amaranth Crunch with Raisins *(Health Valley)*	★
Amaranth Flakes *(Health Valley)*	★
Amaranth with Bananas *(Health Valley)*	★
Amaranth, Blueberry *(Good Shepherd)*	★
Arrowhead Crunch *(Arrowhead Mills)*	★
Banana Pecan, Breakfast Cup *(Casbah)*	4
Barley Plus *(Erewhon)*	★
Barley, Quick *(Quaker)*	★
Bear Mush *(Arrowhead Mills)*	★
Blue Corn Flakes *(Health Valley)*	★
Blueberry Cup, Breakfast Cup *(Casbah)*	4
Bran Buds *(Kellogg's)*	2 3
Bran Flakes *(Arrowhead Mills)*	★
Bran Flakes *(Kellogg's)*	2
Bran Flakes *(Post)*	2
Bran Flakes *(Stone-Buhr)*	★
Breakfast Biscuits *(Barbara's)*	★
Breakfast O's *(Barbara's)*	★
Brown Rice *(Grainfield's)*	★
Brown Rice Cream *(Erewhon)*	★
Brown Rice Crisps *(Barbara's)*	2
Brown Rice, Crispy *(Erewhon)*	2
Brown Rice, Crispy *(New Morning)*	★
Brown Rice, Crispy - Low Sodium *(Erewhon)*	★
Bulgur Wheat *(Arrowhead Mills)*	★
Bulgur Wheat with Soy Grits *(Hodgson Mill)*	★
C. W. Post *(Post)*	★
Cherrios *(General Mills)*	2
Cherrios, Honey Nut *(General Mills)*	2 3
Corn & Amaranth, Aztec *(Erewhon)*	★
Corn Flakes *(Arrowhead Mills)*	★
Corn Flakes *(Barbara's)*	2

1 = High Fat   2 = High Sodium   3 = High Refined Sugar   5 = Cholesterol
1+ = Very High Fat   2+ = Very High Sodium   4 = Highly Processed   ★= Better Choice

VARIETY *(Brand)*   RATING CODE

VARIETY (Brand)	★	1	2	3	4
Corn Flakes *(Grainfield's)*	★				
Corn Flakes *(New Morning)*	★				
Corn Flakes, Honey Frosted *(New Morning)*				3	
Corn Grits, White *(Arrowhead Mills)*	★				
Corn Grits, Yellow *(Arrowhead Mills)*	★				
Cracked Wheat *(Arrowhead Mills)*	★				
Cracked Wheat *(Hodgson Mill)*	★				
Cracked Wheat *(Stone-Buhr)*	★				
Cream of Rice *(Nabisco)*					4
Cream of Rye *(Roman Meal)*				3	
Cream of Wheat, Instant *(Nabisco)*					4
Cream of Wheat, Regular *(Nabisco)*					4
Crispy Oats *(Kölln)*	★				
Crispy Wheats 'n Raisins *(General Mills)*	★				
Crunchy Cereal, Honey Almond *(Northern Gold)*		1		3	
Fiber 7 Flakes *(Health Valley)*	★				
5-Grain *(American Prairie)*	★				
4-Grain Cereal + Flax *(Arrowhead Mills)*	★				
4-Grain Cereal Mates *(Stone-Buhr)*	★				
14 Grains, Hot Cereal *(Barbara's)*	★				
Fruit & Fitness *(Health Valley)*	★				
Fruit 'n Oat Bran Crunch *(Kölln)*	★				
Fruit 'n Wheat *(Erewhon)*			2		
Fruit Lites, Corn *(Health Valley)*	★				
Fruit Lites, Rice *(Health Valley)*	★				
Fruit Lites, Wheat *(Health Valley)*	★				
Fruit-e-O's *(New Morning)*	★				
Graham Flakes, Crispy *(Healthy Times)*	★				
Granola with Bran *(Erewhon)*		1		3	
Granola, Almond Raisin *(The Bread Shop)*		1			
Granola, Apple Amaranth *(Arrowhead Mills)*				3	
Granola, Banana Almond *(Little Debbie)*				3	
Granola, Banana Almond *(Sunbelt)*	★				

1 = High Fat   2 = High Sodium   3 = High Refined Sugar   5 = Cholesterol
1+ = Very High Fat   2+ = Very High Sodium   4 = Highly Processed   ★= Better Choice

VARIETY *(Brand)*   RATING CODE

VARIETY (Brand)				
Granola, Blueberry 'n Cream *(The Bread Shop)*	1			
Granola, Branana Oat Bran *(The Bread Shop)*	1			
Granola, California Orange Crunch *(The Bread Shop)*	1	3		
Granola, Cinnapple Spice *(The Bread Shop)*	1	3		
Granola, Crunchy Oat Bran *(The Bread Shop)*	1			
Granola, Date Nut *(Erewhon)*	1	3		
Granola, Fruit & Nut *(Little Debbie)*	1	3		
Granola, Golden Maple Nut *(The Bread Shop)*	1	3		
Granola, Gone Nuts! *(The Bread Shop)*	1			
Granola, Honey Almond *(Erewhon)*	1	3		
Granola, Honey Almond *(Food for Health)*	1	3		
Granola, Honey Apple Blueberry *(The Bread Shop)*	1	3		
Granola, Honey Gone Nuts! *(The Bread Shop)*	1	3		
Granola, Maple *(Erewhon)*	1	3		
Granola, Maple Nut *(Arrowhead Mills)*	1	3		
Granola, Maple Nut *(Food for Health)*	1	3		
Granola, Oat Bran *(Golden Temple)*	★			
Granola, Oat Bran with Raisins *(The Bread Shop)*	1			
Granola, Orange Almond *(The Bread Shop)*	1			
Granola, Oregon Blueberry Crunch *(The Bread Shop)*	1	3		
Granola, Peaches 'n Cream *(The Bread Shop)*	1			
Granola, Raspberries 'n Cream *(The Bread Shop)*	1			
Granola, Spiced Apple *(Erewhon)*	1	3		
Granola, Strawberries 'n Cream *(The Bread Shop)*	1			
Granola, Sunflower Crunch *(Erewhon)*		3		
Granola, Super Cereal *(The Bread Shop)*	1	3		
Granola, Supernatural *(The Bread Shop)*	1	3		
Grape-Nuts *(Post)*		2		
Grape-Nuts Flakes *(Post)*		2		
Grape-Nuts, Raisin *(Post)*	★			
Grits, Quick *(Quaker)*			4	
Grits, Quick White *(Dixie Lily)*			4	
Grits, White Pearl Hominy *(Dixie Lily)*			4	

1 = High Fat	2 = High Sodium	3 = High Refined Sugar	5 = Cholesterol
1+ = Very High Fat	2+ = Very High Sodium	4 = Highly Processed	★= Better Choice

VARIETY *(Brand)*   RATING CODE

Variety (Brand)	★	2	3	4
Grits, Yellow *(Dixie Lily)*				4
Healthy Crunch, Almond Date *(Health Valley)*	★			
Healthy Crunch, Apple Cinnamon *(Health Valley)*	★			
Healthy O's *(Health Valley)*	★			
Heartland *(Heartland)*			3	
Heartland with Raisins *(Heartland)*			3	
Instant Oat Bran, Raisin *(3-Minute)*	★			
Instant Oats & Bran *(3-Minute)*	★			
Kashi, 5 Bran *(Kashi)*	★			
Kix *(General Mills)*		2		
Malt-O-Meal, plus 40% Oat Bran *(Malt-O-Meal)*				4
Malt-O-Meal, Quick *(Malt-O-Meal)*				4
Manna Golden Cereal *(Stone-Buhr)*	★			
Maple Raisin Oats *(American Prairie)*			3	
Müesli *(Alpen)*	★			
Müesli *(Kentaur)*	★			
Müesli, Maple Nut *(New Morning)*	★			
Müesli, Original *(familia)*			3	
Müesli, Original, No Sugar *(familia)*	★			
Müesli, Sweetened *(Kentaur)*			3	
Müesli, Wheat Free *(American Prairie)*	★			
Müesli, Whole Grain *(American Prairie)*	★			
Nature O's *(Arrowhead Mills)*	★			
NutriGrain Almond & Raisins *(Kellogg's)*		2		
NutriGrain Biscuits *(Kellogg's)*	★			
NutriGrain Nuggets *(Kellogg's)*	★			
NutriGrain Raisin Bran *(Kellogg's)*		2		
NutriGrain Wheat *(Kellogg's)*		2		
NutriGrain Wheat & Raisin *(Kellogg's)*	★			
Oat Bran *(Arrowhead Mills)*	★			
Oat Bran *(Hodgson Mill)*	★			
Oat Bran *(Mother's)*	★			
Oat Bran *(Nabisco)*	★			

1 = High Fat	2 = High Sodium	3 = High Refined Sugar	5 = Cholesterol
1+ = Very High Fat	2+ = Very High Sodium	4 = Highly Processed	★= Better Choice

VARIETY *(Brand)*   RATING CODE

Oat Bran *(New Morning)*	★		
Oat Bran *(Quaker)*	★		
Oat Bran *(Skinners)*	★		
Oat Bran Crunch *(Edward & Sons)*	★		
Oat Bran Flakes *(Arrowhead Mills)*	★		
Oat Bran Flakes *(Health Valley)*	★		
Oat Bran Flakes & Raisins *(Health Valley)*	★		
Oat Bran Flakes, Almonds & Dates *(Health Valley)*	★		
Oat Bran Flakes, Ultimate *(New Morning)*	★		
Oat Bran Hot Cereal, Apple & Cinnamon *(Health Valley)*	★		
Oat Bran Hot Cereal, Raisin & Spice *(Health Valley)*	★		
Oat Bran O's *(Health Valley)*	★		
Oat Bran O's, Fruit & Nut *(Health Valley)*	★		
Oat Bran, 100% Crunchy Oat, Blueberry *(Barbara's)*	★		
Oat Bran, 100% Crunchy Oat, Plain *(Barbara's)*	★		
Oat Bran, 100% Crunchy Oat, with Raisins *(Barbara's)*	★		
Oat Bran, Almond Crunch *(Health Valley)*	★		
Oat Bran, Apple Cinnamon *(Hodgson Mill)*	★		
Oat Bran, Hawaiian Fruit *(Health Valley)*	★		
Oat Bran, Honey Instant *(Nabisco)*		2	3
Oat Bran, Instant *(Nabisco)*	★		
Oat Bran, Instant *(3-Minute)*	★		
Oat Bran, Maple & Brown Sugar *(Hodgson Mill)*	★		
Oat Bran, Natural *(3-Minute)*	★		
Oat Bran, Raisin Nut *(Health Valley)*	★		
Oat Bran, Regular, Instant *(Nabisco)*	★		
Oat Bran, with Wheat Germ *(Erewhon)*	★		
Oatios *(New Morning)*	★		
Oatios, Honey Almond *(New Morning)*			3
Oatmeal *(Edward & Sons)*	★		
Oatmeal, Apple Cinnamon *(Erewhon)*	★		
Oatmeal, Apple Raisin *(Erewhon)*	★		
Oatmeal, Instant *(Arrowhead Mills)*	★		

1 = High Fat	2 = High Sodium	3 = High Refined Sugar	5 = Cholesterol
1+ = Very High Fat	2+ = Very High Sodium	4 = Highly Processed	★= Better Choice

VARIETY *(Brand)*   RATING CODE

Oatmeal, Instant *(Mother's)*	★		
Oatmeal, Instant, Cinnamon & Spice *(Quaker)*		2	3
Oatmeal, Instant, Maple & Brown Sugar *(Quaker)*		2	3
Oatmeal, Instant, Oat Bran Regular Flavor *(3-Minute)*		2	
Oatmeal, Instant, Regular Flavor *(Quaker)*		2	
Oatmeal, Maple Spice *(Erewhon)*	★		
Oatmeal, Old-Fashioned *(Quaker)*	★		
Oatmeal, Old-Fashioned *(3-Minute)*	★		
Oatmeal, Old-Fashioned, Oat Bran *(3-Minute)*	★		
Oatmeal, Quick *(Quaker)*	★		
Oatmeal, Quick *(3-Minute)*	★		
Oatmeal, Quick, Oat Bran *(3-Minute)*	★		
Oatmeal, Quick, Pan Toasted *(3-Minute)*	★		
Oatmeal, Raisin Oats *(3-Minute)*	★		
Oatmeal, Raisins, Dates & Walnuts *(Erewhon)*	★		
Oatmeal, with added Oat Bran *(Erewhon)*	★		
Oats, Crystal Wedding *(Quaker)*	★		
Oats, Quick *(New Morning)*	★		
Oats, Steel Cut *(Arrowhead Mills)*	★		
Oats, Wheat, Dates, Raisins, Almonds *(Roman Meal)*	★		
Oats, Wheat, Rye, Bran, Flax *(Roman Meal)*	★		
Old-Fashioned Rolled Oats *(Stone-Buhr)*	★		
Old-Fashioned Rye Flakes *(Stone-Duhr)*	★		
100% Bran *(Nabisco)*		2	3
100% Natural Bran with Apples & Cinnamon *(Health Valley)*	★		
100% Natural Bran with Raisins & Spice *(Health Valley)*	★		
Orangeola, Almonds & Dates *(Health Valley)*	★		
Orangeola, Bananas & Hawaiian Fruit *(Health Valley)*	★		
Puffed Corn *(Arrowhead Mills)*	★		
Puffed Corn *(Health Valley)*	★		
Puffed Kashi *(Kashi)*	★		
Puffed Millet *(Arrowhead Mills)*	★		
Puffed Rice *(Arrowhead Mills)*	★		

1 = High Fat	2 = High Sodium	3 = High Refined Sugar	5 = Cholesterol
1+ = Very High Fat	2+ = Very High Sodium	4 = Highly Processed	★= Better Choice

VARIETY *(Brand)* — RATING CODE

Variety (Brand)	★	1	2	3	4
Puffed Rice *(Health Valley)*	★				
Puffed Rice *(Popeye)*					4
Puffed Wheat *(Arrowhead Mills)*	★				
Puffed Wheat *(Health Valley)*	★				
Puffed Wheat *(Malt-O-Meal)*					4
Puffed Wheat *(Quaker)*	★				
Quick Cooked Rolled Oats *(Stone-Buhr)*	★				
Raisin Bran *(Barbara's)*	★				
Raisin Bran *(Erewhon)*	★				
Raisin Bran *(Grainfield's)*	★				
Raisin Bran *(Kellogg's)*			2		
Raisin Bran *(New Morning)*	★				
Raisin Bran *(Post)*			2		
Raisin Bran *(Skinner's)*	★				
Raisin Bran Flakes *(Health Valley)*	★				
Raisin Hazelnut, Breakfast Cup *(Casbah)*					4
Raisin Oats Plus Oat Bran *(3-Minute)*	★				
Raspberry Nut, Breakfast Cup *(Casbah)*					4
Rice & Shine *(Arrowhead Mills)*	★				
Rice Bran *(Gourmet Award)*		1+			
Rice Bran Honey Crunch *(Quaker)*				3	
Rice Bran O's *(Health Valley)*	★				
Rice Bran, Almonds & Dates *(Health Valley)*	★				
Rice, Creamy *(Lundberg)*	★				
Scotch Oats *(Stone-Buhr)*	★				
Seven Grain *(Arrowhead Mills)*	★				
7-Grain Cereal *(Stone-Buhr)*	★				
Sprouts, 7, Banana, Hawaiian *(Health Valley)*	★				
Sprouts, 7, Raisin *(Health Valley)*	★				
Stoned Wheat Flakes *(Health Valley)*	★				
Sun Country Granola, Almonds *(Quaker)*		1			
Super Bran *(New Morning)*	★				
Super O's *(Erewhon)*	★				

1 = High Fat 2 = High Sodium 3 = High Refined Sugar 5 = Cholesterol
1+ = Very High Fat 2+ = Very High Sodium 4 = Highly Processed ★= Better Choice

VARIETY *(Brand)*   RATING CODE

Variety (Brand)	★	1	3	
Swiss Breakfast, Raisin Nut *(Health Valley)*	★			
Swiss Breakfast, Tropical Fruit *(Health Valley)*	★			
Uncle Sam *(US Mills)*	★			
Weetabix *(Weetabix)*	★			
Wheat Bran *(Arrowhead Mills)*	★			
Wheat Bran *(Hodgson Mill)*	★			
Wheat Bran, Toasted *(Kretschmer)*		1		
Wheat Flakes *(Arrowhead Mills)*	★			
Wheat Flakes *(Erewhon)*	★			
Wheat Flakes *(Grainfield's)*	★			
Wheat Germ *(Arrowhead Mills)*	★			
Wheat Germ *(Hodgson Mill)*	★			
Wheat Germ *(Kretschmer)*	★			
Wheat Germ, Honey *(Kretschmer)*			3	
Wheat Germ, Untoasted *(Hodgson Mill)*	★			
Wheatena *(Wheatena)*	★			
Whole Millet *(Arrowhead Mills)*	★			
Whole Wheat *(Mother's)*	★			
Whole Wheat Hot Cereal *(Quaker)*	★			

1 = High Fat   2 = High Sodium   3 = High Refined Sugar   5 = Cholesterol
1+ = Very High Fat   2+ = Very High Sodium   4 = Highly Processed   ★= Better Choice

CHEESES

Many cheeses look like a Christmas tree under the rating code with ratings of (1+), (2+), (4) and (5) showing up quite often. This is simply the way *The Food Bible* tells us to limit a food's use — and cheese is no exception. In addition, many cheeses did not make *The Food Bible* because of artificial colors. To muddy the water even more, many processed cheeses contain aluminum to make them softer and more spreadable, and many sliced varieties contain aluminum so they will melt and look prettier on a hamburger. Manufacturers are not required to identify which cheeses have aluminum added, so I was unable to eliminate these from *The Food Bible*. However, I have found through personal testing that the processed varieties and some grated parmesans are the most suspect.

So what are we cheese lovers to do? Personally, I enjoy cheese — the natural kind. I do not care for the taste or texture of processed cheeses. Maybe I have developed this taste after realizing what is in so many of the processed kinds. My favorite cheese is a low-moisture, part skim mozzarella. I will use another cheese once in a while, but it is a rarity. Mozzarella, the low-moisture, part skim, has less fat and cholesterol than any other natural cheese. I rarely use cream cheeses as they are the highest in fat of all the cheeses. They should definitely be limited.

Most cottage cheese is processed locally and marketed under a local brand. Therefore, we do not have many national brands; however, its cousin, ricotta cheese, is distributed nationally. Cottage cheese and ricotta cheese can be good sources of lowfat protein — that is, if the product contains less than 2% butterfat. Unfortunately, when fat is reduced, many times the sodium is increased.

Our best choice is under 2% butterfat and no salt. If the no-salt is not available, let me share a trick with you. Place cottage or ricotta cheese in a strainer and allow water to run through it for a few seconds. This process will rinse away most of the salt. Nearly all brands of cottage and ricotta cheese are free of additives and preservatives. I rate these cheeses as two of our better dairy choices — if they are lowfat.

VARIETY *(Brand)*   RATING CODE

CHEESES
CHEESES, CHEESE

Variety (Brand)				
American Flavor *(Weight Watchers)*	1	2+	4	
American Flavor, Low Sodium *(Weight Watchers)*	1	2	4	
American Singles *(Kraft)*	1+	2+	4	5
American Singles, Deluxe *(Kraft)*	1+	2+	4	5
American Singles, Extra Thick *(Kraft)*	1+	2+	4	5
American White *(Alpine Lace)*	1+	2		
Blue Cheese *(Treasure Cave)*	1+	2+		5
Blue Cheese, Crumblers *(Kraft)*	1+	2+		5
Bonbel *(The Laughing Cow)*	1+	2		5
Brie *(Corneville)*	1+	2		5
Chedarella *(Lake to Lake)*	1+	2		5
Cheddar *(Alpine Lace)*	1+			5
Cheddar *(Land-O-Lakes)*	1+	2		5
Cheddar *(Tillamook)*	1+	2		5
Cheddar, 40% Less *(Weight Watchers)*	1+	2	4	
Cheddar, Extra Sharp *(Kraft)*	1+	2		5
Cheddar, Extra Sharp *(Tillamook)*	1+	2		5
Cheddar, Golden Image *(Kraft)*	1+	2	4	
Cheddar, Lite, Shredded *(Frigo)*	1+	2	4	
Cheddar, Longhorn *(Lake to Lake)*	1+	2		5
Cheddar, Medium *(Tillamook)*	1+	2		5
Cheddar, Medium, Mild & Sharp Slices *(Kraft)*	1+	2		5
Cheddar, Mild *(County Line)*	1+	2		5
Cheddar, Mild *(Dakota Farms)*	1+	2		5
Cheddar, Mild *(Kraft)*	1+	2		5
Cheddar, Mild *(Lake to Lake)*	1+	2		5
Cheddar, Mild *(Wisconsin's Famous)*	1+	2	4	
Cheddar, Mild Flavor *(Weight Watchers)*	1+	2	4	
Cheddar, Mild Longhorn Style *(Kraft)*	1+	2		5
Cheddar, Mild, Medium, Sharp, Extra Sharp *(Harvest Moon)*	1+	2		5
Cheddar, Mild, Mootown Snackers *(Sargento)*	1+			5
Cheddar, Mild, Shredded *(Kraft)*	1+	2		5
Cheddar, Mild, Shredded *(Sargento)*	1+	2		5

VARIETY (Brand) — RATING CODE

VARIETY (Brand)	Fat	Sodium	Processed	Cholesterol
Cheddar, Sharp (Cache Valley)	1+	2		5
Cheddar, Sharp (Kraft)	1+	2		5
Cheddar, Sharp (Lake to Lake)	1+	2		5
Cheddar, Sharp (Tillamook)	1+	2		5
Cheddar, Sharp Flavor (Weight Watchers)	1+	2	4	
Cheddar, Sharp Flavor Singles (Weight Watchers)	1	2+	4	
Cheddar, Sharp, Mootown Snackers (Sargento)	1+	2		5
Cheddar, Sharp, Shredded (Kraft)	1+	2		5
Cheddar, Sharp, Shredded (Sargento)	1+	2		5
Cheddar, Shredded (County Line)	1+	2		5
Cheddar, Shredded (Frigo)	1+	2		5
Cheddar, Shredded (Lakeshire)	1+	2		5
Cheddar, Sliced (Lucerne)	1+	2		5
Colbi-Lo (Alpine Lace)	1+			5
Colby (Dakota Farms)	1+	2		5
Colby (Land-O-Lakes)	1+	2		5
Colby Flavor (Weight Watchers)	1+	2	4	
Colby, Jack (County Line)	1+	2		5
Colby, Longhorn (Lake to Lake)	1+	2		5
Colby, Longhorn Style (Kraft)	1+	2		5
Colby, Mild (Kraft)	1+	2		5
Colby, Monterey Jack (Kraft)	1+	2		5
Colby, Monterey Jack, Shredded (Kraft)	1+	2		5
Colby, Sharp (Dakota Farms)	1+	2		5
Colby, Slices (Kraft)	1+	2		5
Colby-Jack Longhorn (Cache Valley)	1+	2		5
Colby-Jack, Mootown Snackers (Sargento)	1+	2		5
Colby-Jack, Shredded (Sargento)	1+	2		5
Cold Pack Blue Cheese (Kraft)	1+	2+		5
Cottage Cheese (Alta•Dena)	1+	2+		
Cottage Cheese, 1% (Weight Watchers)		2+		
Cottage Cheese, 1%, No Salt (Lucerne)	★			
Cottage Cheese, 2% (Borden)		2+		

1 = High Fat   2 = High Sodium   3 = High Refined Sugar   5 = Cholesterol
1+ = Very High Fat   2+ = Very High Sodium   4 = Highly Processed   ★= Better Choice

VARIETY *(Brand)*   RATING CODE

Variety (Brand)	Rating Code		
Cottage Cheese, 2% *(Lucerne)*		2+	
Cottage Cheese, 4% *(Borden)*	1	2+	
Cottage Cheese, 4% *(Lucerne)*	1	2+	
Cottage Cheese, Dry Curd *(Lucerne)*	★		
Cottage Cheese, Lowfat *(Alta·Dena)*		2+	
Cracker Barrel, Baby Swiss *(Kraft)*	1+		5
Cracker Barrel, Cheddar *(Kraft)*	1+	2	5
Cracker Barrel, Extra Sharp *(Kraft)*	1+	2	5
Cracker Barrel, Extra Sharp Cheddar *(Kraft)*	1+	2	5
Cracker Barrel, Gouda *(Kraft)*	1+	2+	5
Cracker Barrel, Havarti *(Kraft)*	1+		5
Cracker Barrel, Muenster *(Kraft)*	1+	2	5
Cracker Barrel, Sharp *(Kraft)*	1+	2	5
Cracker Barrel, Sharp Cheddar *(Kraft)*	1+	2	5
Cracker Barrel, Vermont Sharp White *(Kraft)*	1+	2	5
Edam *(Kraft)*	1+	2	5
Edam *(Kaukauna)*	1+	2	5
Edam *(May-Bud)*	1+	2+	5
Edam *(Sargento)*	1+	2+	5
Edam *(The Laughing Cow)*	1+	2+	5
Edam *(White Clover Dairy)*	1+	2	5
Farmer's *(May-Bud)*	1+		5
Farmer's *(Sargento)*	1+		5
Farmer's *(The Laughing Cow)*	1+		5
Feta *(Athenos)*	1+	2+	5
Feta *(Treasure Cave)*	1+	2+	5
Feta *(Vigo)*	1+	2+	5
Fontinella *(Stella)*	1+	2	5
Gouda *(Kaukauna)*	1+	2	5
Gouda *(Kraft)*	1+		5
Gouda *(May-Bud)*	1+	2	5
Gouda *(White Clover Dairy)*	1+	2	5
Italian Blend, Grated *(Kraft)*	1+	2+	5

1 = High Fat   2 = High Sodium   3 = High Refined Sugar   5 = Cholesterol
1+ = Very High Fat   2+ = Very High Sodium   4 = Highly Processed   ★= Better Choice

VARIETY *(Brand)*   RATING CODE

Italian Style, Grated *(Sargento)*	1+	2+		5
Light & Lively, American *(Kraft)*	1+	2+	4	
Light Natural Cheddar *(Kraft)*	1+	2	4	5
Light Natural Cheddar, Shredded *(Kraft)*	1+	2	4	5
Light Natural Colby *(Kraft)*	1+	2	4	5
Light Natural Monterey Jack *(Kraft)*	1+	2	4	5
Light Natural Swiss *(Kraft)*	1		4	
Light Natural Swiss, Low Sodium *(Kraft)*	1+		4	5
Light Natural, Low Sodium *(Kraft)*	1+		4	5
Limburger *(Mohawk Valley)*	1+	2		5
Lite-Line, Swiss *(Borden)*	1+	2+	4	
Monterey Jack *(Casino)*	1+	2		5
Monterey Jack *(Dakota Farms)*	1+	2		5
Monterey Jack *(General Store)*	1+	2		5
Monterey Jack *(Harvest Moon)*	1+	2		5
Monterey Jack *(Lake to Lake)*	1+	2		5
Monterey Jack *(Lakeshire)*	1+	2		5
Monterey Jack *(May-Bud)*	1+	2		5
Monterey Jack *(Weight Watchers)*	1+	2	4	
Monterey Jack *(Wisconsin's Finest)*	1+	2	4	
Monterey Jack Slices *(Kraft)*	1+	2		5
Monterey Jack with Jalapeño *(Casino)*	1+	2		5
Monterey Jack, Shredded *(Kraft)*	1+	2		5
Monti-Jack-Lo *(Alpine Lace)*	1+			
Mozzarella Flavor *(Weight Watchers)*	1+	2	4	
Mozzarella, LM/PS * *(Alpine Lace)*	1+	2		
Mozzarella, LM/PS * *(Casino)*	1+	2		
Mozzarella, LM/PS * *(Frigo)*	1+			
Mozzarella, LM/PS * *(General Store)*	1+	2		5
Mozzarella, LM/PS * *(Harvest)*	1+	2		
Mozzarella, LM/PS * *(Lakeshire)*	1+	2		
Mozzarella, LM/PS * *(Precious)*	1+			
Mozzarella, LM/PS * *(Sargento)*	1+	2		

*LM/PS = Low Moisture/Part Skim

1 = High Fat	2 = High Sodium	3 = High Refined Sugar	5 = Cholesterol
1+ = Very High Fat	2+ = Very High Sodium	4 = Highly Processed	★= Better Choice

VARIETY *(Brand)*   RATING CODE

Variety (Brand)	1	1+	2	2+	4	5	★
Mozzarella, LM/PS * *(Wisconsin's Finest)*		1+	2				
Mozzarella, Shredded, LM/PS * *(County Line)*		1+	2				
Mozzarella, Shredded, LM/PS * *(Frigo)*		1+	2				
Mozzarella, Shredded, LM/PS * *(Kraft)*		1+	2				
Mozzarella, Shredded, LM/PS * *(Lucerne)*		1+	2				
Mozzarella, Shredded, LM/PS * *(Sargento)*		1+	2				
Mozzarella, Shredded, LM/PS * *(Wisconsin's Finest)*		1+	2				
Mozzarella, Slices, LM/PS * *(Kraft)*		1+	2				
Mozzarella, Whole Milk *(Maggio)*		1+		2+		5	
Mozzarella, Whole Milk *(Polly-O)*		1+	2			5	
Muenster *(Alpine)*		1+	2			5	
Muenster *(Cache Valley)*		1+	2			5	
Muenster, Queso Blanco *(Sargento)*		1+	2			5	
Old English Loaf *(Kraft)*		1+		2+	4	5	
Parmesan *(Kraft)*		1+		2+		5	
Parmesan & Romano, Grated *(Sargento)*		1+		2+		5	
Parmesan, Grated *(Sargento)*		1+		2+		5	
Parmesan, Grated - in jar *(Progresso)*		1+		2+		5	
Parmesan, Shredded *(Kraft)*		1+		2+		5	
Parmesan, Shredded *(Sargento)*		1+		2+			
Pepper, Jalapeño *(Kraft)*		1+		2+	4	5	
Pimento Singles *(Kraft)*		1+		2+	4	5	
Pimento Slices *(Kraft)*				2+	4		
Ricotta *(Breakstone's)*		1+				5	
Ricotta *(Miceli's)*		1+				5	
Ricotta, Lite *(Miceli's)*	1					5	
Ricotta, Lite *(Polly-O)*							★
Ricotta, Lite *(Precious)*	1					5	
Ricotta, Lite *(Sargento)*	1					5	
Ricotta, Low Fat, Part Skim *(Maggio)*		1+				5	
Ricotta, Part Skim *(Axelrod)*		1+				5	
Ricotta, Part Skim *(Polly-O)*		1+				5	
Ricotta, Part Skim *(Precious)*		1+				5	

*LM/PS = Low Moisture/Part Skim

1 = High Fat	2 = High Sodium	3 = High Refined Sugar	5 = Cholesterol
1+ = Very High Fat	2+ = Very High Sodium	4 = Highly Processed	★= Better Choice

VARIETY (Brand) — RATING CODE

VARIETY (Brand)				
Ricotta, Part Skim (Sargento)	1+			5
Ricotta, Whole Milk (Axelrod)	1+			5
Ricotta, Whole Milk (Maggio)	1+			5
Ricotta, Whole Milk (Polly-O)	1+			5
Ricotta, Whole Milk (Precious)	1+			5
Ricotta, Whole Milk (Sorrento)	1+			5
Romano, Grated (Kraft)	1+	2+		5
String Cheddar, LM/PS * (Kraft)	1+	2		
String Mozzarella, LM/PS * (Baker)	1+	2		5
String Mozzarella, LM/PS * (County Line)	1+	2		
String Mozzarella, LM/PS * (Frigo)	1+	2		
String Mozzarella, LM/PS * (Kraft)	1+	2		
String Mozzarella, LM/PS * (Sargento)	1+	2		
String Mozzarella, LM/PS * (Sorrento)	1+	2		
Swiss (Lake to Lake)	1+	2		5
Swiss Flavor (Weight Watchers)	1		4	
Swiss Singles (Kraft)	1+	2+	4	
Swiss, Shredded (Kraft)	1+			5
Swiss, Slices (Kraft)	1+			
Swiss-Lo (Alpine Lace)	1+			5
Swisson Rye (Hoffman's)	1+	2+	4	5
Velvetta (Kraft)	1+	2+	4	5
Velvetta, Extra Thick Slices (Kraft)	1+	2+	4	5
Velvetta, Hot Mexican (Kraft)	1+	2+	4	5
Velvetta, Mexican, Shredded (Kraft)	1+	2+	4	5
Velvetta, Mild Mexican (Kraft)	1+	2+	4	5
Velvetta, Shredded (Kraft)	1+	2+	4	5
Velvetta, Slices (Kraft)	1+	2+	4	5
CHEESES: SOFT CHEESE				
Country Crock, Cheddar (Shedd's)	1+	2	4	
Country Crock, Herb & Garlic (Shedd's)	1+	2	4	
Country Crock, Mexican (Shedd's)	1+	2	4	

*LM/PS = Low Moisture/Part Skim

1 = High Fat   2 = High Sodium   3 = High Refined Sugar   5 = Cholesterol
1+ = Very High Fat   2+ = Very High Sodium   4 = Highly Processed   ★ = Better Choice

VARIETY *(Brand)*   RATING CODE

Variety (Brand)			
Cream Cheese *(Fleur-de-Lait)*	1+		5
Cream Cheese, Light *(Philadelphia)*	1+		5
Cream Cheese, Soft *(Philadelphia)*	1+		5
Cream Cheese, Soft Chives & Onion *(Philadelphia)*	1+		5
Cream Cheese, Soft Herb & Garlic *(Philadelphia)*	1+ 2		5
Cream Cheese, Soft Light *(Philadelphia)*	1+ 2		5
Cream Cheese, Soft Pineapple *(Philadelphia)*	1+		5
Extra Sharp Cheddar *(Kaukauna)*	1+ 2+	4	5
Hearty Horseradish *(Kaukauna)*	1+ 2+	4	5
Olive & Pimento Spread *(Kraft)*	1+ 2	4	
Pimento Spread *(Kraft)*	1+ 2	4	
Pineapple Spread *(Kraft)*	1+	4	
Sharp Cheddar *(Kaukauna)*	1+ 2+	4	5
Sharp Cheddar *(Wispride)*	1+ 2+	4	5
Spreadery, French Onion *(Kraft)*	1+ 2	4	5
Spreadery, Garden Vegetables *(Kraft)*	1+ 2+	4	5
Spreadery, Garlic & Herb *(Kraft)*	1+ 2	4	5
Spreadery, Medium Cheddar *(Kraft)*	1+ 2+	4	
Spreadery, Mexican *(Kraft)*	1+ 2+	4	
Spreadery, Mild Cheddar *(Kraft)*	1+ 2+	4	
Swiss Almond *(Kaukauna)*	1+ 2+	4	5
Swiss Almond *(Scott's)*	1+ 2+	4	5
Velvetta Cheese Sauce, Mexican Micro *(Kraft)*	1+ 2+	4	5
Velvetta Cheese Sauce, Micro *(Kraft)*	1+ 2+	4	5

1 = High Fat   2 = High Sodium   3 = High Refined Sugar   5 = Cholesterol
1+ = Very High Fat   2+ = Very High Sodium   4 = Highly Processed   ★= Better Choice

CONDIMENTS AND MISCELLANEOUS

I cannot classify most items listed here as food; however, most add unique flavors to foods. The biggest item to watch is the sodium content — which can be very high. Fortunately, we generally do not eat condiments in large portions. Most condiments not included in *The Food Bible* contain sodium benzoate or potassium bromate, and most all pickled products contain polysorbates and artificial colors, including yellow #5.

I personally do not use a lot of condiments, but when I do, I like those with zip, such as horseradish, mustard, etc.

As for olives, they are naturally high in fat. Also, quite a bit of salt is used in canning; so this food has two strikes against it. Most all green olives did not make *The Food Bible* because of sodium alginate. Black olives normally do not contain additives or preservatives. As a group, I do not rate olives very high. They contain a lot of fat and salt, and very few nutrients. As a food, we do not need them; so it is best to limit their consumption.

VARIETY *(Brand)*   RATING CODE

CONDIMENTS AND MISCELLANEOUS
CONDIMENTS

Capers *(Amico)*	2+
Capers *(Del Rio)*	2+
Capers *(Faraon)*	2+
Catsup *(Hain)*	2+ 3
Catsup *(Town House)*	2+ 3
Catsup, No Salt Added *(Hain)*	3
Chili Sauce *(Bennett's)*	2+ 3
Chili Sauce *(Heinz)*	2+ 3
Chow-Chow, Corn *(Braswell's)*	2+ 3
Chow-Chow, Hot & Mild *(Braswell's)*	2+ 3
Horse Radish *(Schnitzius)*	2+
Horseradish, Creamed & Refrigerated *(Kraft)*	2+
Horseradish, Refrigerated *(Kraft)*	2+
Hot Sauce *(Crystal)*	2+
Hot Sauce *(Louisiana)*	2+
Hot Sauce, Cajun Sunshine *(Try Me)*	2
Hot Sauce, Red Hot *(Durkee)*	2+
Ketchup *(Del Monte)*	2+ 3
Ketchup *(Heinz)*	2+ 3
Ketchup *(Hunt's)*	2+ 3
Ketchup *(Weight Watchers)*	2+ 3
Ketchup, Hot *(Heinz)*	2+ 3
Ketchup, Lite *(Heinz)*	2+ 3
Ketchup, No Salt *(Hunt's)*	3
Louisiana Hot Sauce *(La Preferida)*	2
Maggi Seasoning *(Maggi)*	2+
Marinade *(Allegro)*	2+
Mint Sauce *(Crosse & Blackwell)*	2+ 3
Mustard *(BestYet)*	1 2+
Mustard *(Dusseldorf)*	1 2+
Mustard *(French's)*	1 2+
Mustard *(Garden Club)*	1 2+
Mustard *(Koops')*	1 2+

1 = High Fat 2 = High Sodium 3 = High Refined Sugar 5 = Cholesterol
1+ = Very High Fat 2+ = Very High Sodium 4 = Highly Processed ★= Better Choice

VARIETY *(Brand)*	RATING CODE
Mustard *(Kraft)*	1 2+
Mustard *(Old Monk)*	1 2+
Mustard *(Sauer's)*	1 2+
Mustard, Bavarian Style *(Reese)*	1 2+
Mustard, Bold 'N Spicy *(French's)*	1 2+
Mustard, Country Dijon *(Grey Poupon)*	1 2+
Mustard, Creole *(Luzianne)*	1 2+
Mustard, Dijon *(Coleman)*	1 2+
Mustard, Dijon *(French's)*	1 2+
Mustard, Dijon *(Grey Poupon)*	1 2+
Mustard, Dijon *(Old Monk)*	1 2+
Mustard, Dijon, Squeeze *(Lawry's)*	1 2+
Mustard, Dusseldorf Style *(Reese)*	1 2+
Mustard, Extra Strong *(Pommery)*	1 2+
Mustard, French with Tarragon *(International Bazaar)*	1 2+
Mustard, Golden Dijon 100% Natural *(Lawry's)*	1 2+
Mustard, Horseradish *(French's)*	1 2+
Mustard, Horseradish *(Koops')*	1 2+
Mustard, Horseradish *(Tulkoff)*	1 2+
Mustard, Hot *(Ty Ling)*	1 2+
Mustard, Hot, Chinese Style *(Port Arthur)*	1 2+
Mustard, Hot, Original *(Mister Mustard)*	1 2+
Mustard, Natural *(Plochman's)*	1 2+
Mustard, Original *(Grey Poupon)*	1 2+
Mustard, Parisian *(Grey Poupon)*	1 2+
Mustard, Pommery *(Pommery)*	1 2+
Mustard, Spicy Brown *(Gulden's)*	1 2+
Mustard, Spicy Brown Squeeze Bottle *(Gulden's)*	1 2+
Mustard, Squeeze *(Plochman's)*	1 2+
Mustard, Stadium *(Davis)*	1 2+
Mustard, Stone Ground *(Hain)*	1 2+
Mustard, Stone Ground *(inglehoffer)*	1 2+
Mustard, Stone Ground *(Plochman's)*	1 2+

1 = High Fat 2 = High Sodium 3 = High Refined Sugar 5 = Cholesterol
1+ = Very High Fat 2+ = Very High Sodium 4 = Highly Processed ★= Better Choice

VARIETY *(Brand)*   RATING CODE

Variety (Brand)			
Mustard, Stone Ground, No Salt Added *(Hain)*	1		
Mustard, Sweet Hot *(inglehoffer)*	1	2+	
Mustard, Sweet 'n Hot *(Silver Spring)*	1	2+	
Pickapeppa Sauce *(Pickapeppa)*		2+	3
Seafood Cocktail Sauce *(Heinz)*		2+	3
Seafood Cocktail Sauce *(Reese)*		2+	3
Steak Sauce *(A-1)*		2+	
Steak Sauce *(HP)*	★		
Steak Sauce *(Prime Choice)*		2+	
Sweet 'n Sour *(Sauceworks)*			3
Tabasco *(McIlhenny's)*		2+	
Tartar Sauce, Lite *(Golden Dipt)*	1+	2	3
Tennessee Sunshine *(Try Me)*		2+	
Worcestershire *(French's)*		2+	
Worcestershire *(Lea & Perrins)*		2+	
Worcestershire, Wine & Pepper *(Try Me)*		2+	

FLAVORINGS

Flavorings			
Best o' Butter *(McCormick)*	2+		
Butter Buds *(Butter Buds)*	2+	3	4
Butter Magic, Butter Flavor *(Williams)*	2+	3	4
Molly McButter, Butter Flavor *(Molly McButter)*	2+	3	4
Molly McButter, Cheese *(Molly McButter)*	2+	3	4
Molly McButter, Sour Cream *(Molly McButter)*	2+	3	4

JELLY FIXIN'S

Jelly Fixin's	
Jel 'n Jam *(Kerr)*	3
Jell 'n Jam *(Sure-Jell)*	3
Sure-Jell *(Sure-Jell)*	3
Sure-Jell, Light *(Sure-Jell)*	3

OLIVES, BLACK OLIVES

Olives		
Black Olives *(Del Rio)*	1+	2+
Black Olives *(Mario)*	1+	2+
Black Olives, Amfisse *(Peloponnese)*	1+	2+

1 = High Fat 2 = High Sodium 3 = High Refined Sugar 5 = Cholesterol
1+ = Very High Fat 2+ = Very High Sodium 4 = Highly Processed ★= Better Choice

VARIETY *(Brand)*	RATING CODE
Black Olives, Atalanti *(Peloponnese)*	1+ 2+
Black Olives, Calamata *(Fantis)*	1+ 2+
Black Olives, Calamata *(New Morning)*	1+ 2+
Black Olives, Chopped & Colossal *(Town House)*	1+ 2+
Black Olives, Chopped & Extra Large *(S & W)*	1+ 2+
Black Olives, Chopped, Sliced & Whole *(Durkee)*	1+ 2+
Black Olives, Colossal, Medium & Large *(Vlasic)*	1+ 2+
Black Olives, Extra Large, Pitted *(S & W)*	1+ 2+
Black Olives, Greek *(New Morning)*	1+ 2+
Black Olives, Jumbo *(Reese)*	1+ 2+
Black Olives, Jumbo, Pitted *(S & W)*	1+ 2+
Black Olives, Large & Jumbo *(Early California)*	1+ 2+
Black Olives, Medium California *(Mario)*	1+ 2+
Black Olives, Medium, Pitted *(Gourmet Award)*	1+ 2+
Black Olives, Sliced & Chopped *(Vlasic)*	1+ 2+
Black Olives, Sliced, Jalapeño *(Vlasic)*	1+ 2+
Black Olives, Small, Medium, Large, Chopped *(Lindsay)*	1+ 2+
Black Olives, Small, Medium, Large & Extra Large *(Town House)*	1+ 2+
Black Olives, Small, Medium, Large & Jumbo *(Durkee)*	1+ 2+
OLIVES, GREEN OLIVES	
Green Olives *(Goya)*	1+ 2+
Green Olives *(Mezzetta)*	1+ 2+
Green Olives *(Soleillon)*	1+ 2+
Green Olives with Jalapeño Pepper *(Mezzeta)*	1+ 2+
Green Olives, Almond Stuffed *(Durkee)*	1+ 2+
Green Olives, Almond Stuffed *(Reese)*	1+ 2+
Green Olives, Ionian *(Peloponnese)*	1+ 2+
Green Olives, Jalapeño Stuffed *(Mezzetta)*	1+ 2+
Green Olives, Jalapeño Stuffed *(Spencer)*	1+ 2+
Green Olives, Nafplion *(Peloponnese)*	1+ 2+
Green Olives, Onion Stuffed *(Spencer)*	1+ 2+
Green Olives, Pimento Stuffed *(Spencer)*	1+ 2+

1 = High Fat	2 = High Sodium	3 = High Refined Sugar	5 = Cholesterol
1+ = Very High Fat	2+ = Very High Sodium	4 = Highly Processed	★= Better Choice

VARIETY *(Brand)*　　　　　　　　　RATING CODE

VARIETY (Brand)	Better Choice	Rating
Green Olives, Plain *(Spencer)*		1+ 2+
Green Olives, Plain Queen *(Gourmet Award)*		1+ 2+
Green Olives, Spanish *(New Morning)*		1+ 2+
Green Olives, Texas Spiced *(Spencer)*		1+ 2+
Jalapeño Stuffed Olives *(José Jalapeño)*		1+ 2+
Spanish Olives, Almond Stuffed *(Bella)*		1+ 2+
Spanish Olives, Anchovies *(Bella)*		1+ 2+
Spanish Queen Olives, Pimento *(Mezzetta)*		1+ 2+
Spanish Stuffed Olives *(Durkee)*		1+ 2+
PICKLED FOODS		
Pickle Chips, Honey, No Salt *(New Morning)*		3
Pickled Baby Corn *(Roland)*		2+
Pickled Cocktail Onions *(Durkee)*		2+
Pickled Cocktail Onions *(Gourmet Award)*		2+
Pickled Cornichons *(Reese)*		2+
Pickled Gardiniera *(New Morning)*		2+
Pickled Gardiniera *(Progresso)*		2+
Pickled Pepperoncini *(New Morning)*		2+
Pickled Sweet Cherry Peppers *(Mezzetta)*		2+
Pickles, Dill *(Cascadian Farm)*		2+
Pickles, Dill *(Cosmic)*		2+
Pickles, Dill, Baby *(New Morning)*		2+
Pickles, Dill, Kosher *(New Morning)*		2+
Pickles, Dill, Kosher Spears *(New Morning)*		2+
Pickles, Dill, Kosher, No Salt *(New Morning)*	★	
Pickles, Dill, Spicy Kosher *(Cascadian Farm)*		2+
Pickles, Dill, Spicy Low Sodium *(Cascadian Farm)*		2+
Pickles, Sweet *(Original)*		2+ 3
Relish, Corn, No Salt *(New Morning)*	★	
Relish, Piccalilli, Tomato *(New Morning)*	★	
Relish, Pickle, Sweet *(New Morning)*		3
Relish, Pickle, Sweet, No Sugar *(Pure & Simple)*	★	

1 = High Fat　　2 = High Sodium　　3 = High Refined Sugar　　5 = Cholesterol
1+ = Very High Fat　　2+ = Very High Sodium　　4 = Highly Processed　　★ = Better Choice

COOKIES

Until a year or so ago, most of the cookies I saw in grocery stores were not even food. The nutrients were almost non-existent, and refined sugars, very high fat (most with tropical oils), and additives and preservatives were the norm. This trend seems to be changing somewhat, and more healthful cookies are showing up that can be included in *The Food Bible*.

We still have to watch for additives and preservatives. For example: *Nabisco* Chips Ahoy Sprinkled Cookies have cottonseed oil, artificial flavor, artificial color (yellow #5 and #6), sodium benzoate and potassium sorbate included in their ingredients.

However, on a shelf close by, we'll find *Health Valley* Fat-Free Apricot Delight Cookies, which are an excellent choice with no additives or preservatives and are made with whole grains and no refined sugars. Just stick to *The Food Bible* selections for your best choices.

VARIETY *(Brand)*   RATING CODE

COOKIES

Variety (Brand)			
Almond Butter *(Tree of Life)*	1		
Almond, Toasted *(Barbara's)*	1		
Amaranth *(Health Valley)*	★		
Animal Cookies, Carob *(Barbara's)*	1		
Animal Cookies, Chocolate *(Barbara's)*	1		
Animal Cookies, Cinnamon *(Barbara's)*	1		
Animal Cookies, Ginger Dino Snaps *(Westbrae Natural)*	★		
Animal Cookies, Lemon Dino Snaps *(Westbrae Natural)*	★		
Animal Cookies, Oat Bran *(Health Valley)*	1		
Animal Cookies, Vanilla *(Barbara's)*	1		
Animal Cookies, Vanilla Dino Snaps *(Westbrae Natural)*	1		
Animal Crackers *(Gerber)*		3	4
Animal Frackers *(Frookie)*	1		4
Apple Spice, Fat-Free *(Health Valley)*	★		
Apricot Almond, Fancy Fruit Chunks *(Health Valley)*	1		
Apricot Delight, Fat-Free *(Health Valley)*	★		
Apricot Raspberry Fruit *(Pepperidge Farm)*	1+	3	4
Butter Chessmen *(Pepperidge Farm)*	1+	3	4
Carob Chip *(Tree of Life)*	1		
Carob Fudge *(Tree of Life)*	1		
Carob Snaps *(Westbrae Natural)*	1	3	
Chocolate Chip *(Barbara's)*	1		
Chocolate Chip *(Frookie)*	1		4
Chocolate Chip *(Tree of Life)*	1		
Chocolate Crisps *(Barbara's)*	★		
Chocolate Swirl *(Barbara's)*	1		
Chocolate-Chocolate Chip *(Barbara's)*	1		
Cocoa Chip Snaps *(Westbrae Natural)*	1	3	
Cocoa Snaps *(Westbrae Natural)*	1	3	
Date Delight, Fat-Free *(Health Valley)*	★		
Date Pecan, Fancy Fruit Chunks *(Health Valley)*	1		
Date Walnut *(Barbara's)*	1		
French Vanilla *(Barbara's)*	1		

1 = High Fat   2 = High Sodium   3 = High Refined Sugar   5 = Cholesterol
1+ = Very High Fat   2+ = Very High Sodium   4 = Highly Processed   ★= Better Choice

VARIETY (Brand) — RATING CODE

VARIETY (Brand)			
Fruit & Fitness (Health Valley)	★		
Fruit & Nut (Barbara's)	★		
Fruit & Nut Oat Bran (Health Valley)	1		
Fruit Jumbos, Almond Date (Health Valley)	1		
Fruit Jumbos, Oat Bran (Health Valley)	★		
Fruit Jumbos, Raisin Nut (Health Valley)	1		
Fruit Jumbos, Tropical Fruit (Health Valley)	★		
Fruitins, Apple (Frookie)	★		
Fruitins, Fig (Frookie)	★		
Ginger Snaps (Barbara's)	★		
Ginger Snaps (Westbrae Natural)	1	3	
Ginger Spice (Frookie)	1		4
Graham Crackers, Amaranth (Health Valley)	★		
Graham Crackers, Honey (Health Valley)	1	3	
Graham Crackers, Honey (Mi-Del)		3	
Graham Crackers, Honey (New Morning)		3	
Graham Crackers, Oat Bran (Health Valley)	★		
Honey Jumbos Cinnamon Crisp (Health Valley)		3	
Honey Jumbos Oat Bran (Health Valley)		3	
Honey Jumbos Peanut Butter (Health Valley)		3	
Lemon (Barbara's)	★		
Lemon Snaps (Westbrae Natural)	1	3	
Mandarin Orange Chocolate Chip (Frookie)	1		4
Maple Walnut, Wheat Free (Tree of Life)	1	3	
Mint Chocolate Chip (Frookie)	1		4
Oat Bran Muffin (Frookie)	1		4
Oat Bran, Apple Cinnamon (Frookie)	1		4
Oatmeal (Tree of Life)	1		
Oatmeal Raisin (Barbara's)	★		
Oatmeal Raisin (Frookie)	1		4
Oatmeal Raisin, Wheat Free (Nanak's)	1		
Oatmeal Snaps (Westbrae Natural)	1	3	
Orange (Barbara's)	★		

1 = High Fat   2 = High Sodium   3 = High Refined Sugar   5 = Cholesterol
1+ = Very High Fat   2+ = Very High Sodium   4 = Highly Processed   ★= Better Choice

VARIETY *(Brand)*   RATING CODE

Peanut Butter *(Barbara's)*	1+		
Peanut Butter *(Natures Warehouse)*	1		
Peanut Butter *(Tree of Life)*	1		
Peanut Butter Snaps *(Westbrae Natural)*	1+	3	
Peanut Butter, Wheat Free *(Tree of Life)*	1	3	
Peanut Chunks *(Health Valley)*	2+		
Quinoa Oat Bran, Wheat Free *(Nanak's)*	1		
Raisin Oat Bran, Fancy Fruit Chunks *(Health Valley)*	★		
Raisin Oatmeal, Fat-Free *(Health Valley)*	★		
Rice Applesauce, Wheat Free *(Tree of Life)*	1	3	
Rice Bran *(Tree of Life)*	1		
7-Grain Oatmeal *(Frookie)*	1		4
Strawberry Fruit *(Pepperidge Farm)*	1	3	4
Tofu Cookies *(Health Valley)*	★		
Tropical Fruit, Fancy Fruit Chunks *(Health Valley)*	1		
Vanilla Crisps *(Barbara's)*	★		
Wheat Free Cookie *(Health Valley)*	★		
Wheat Free, Oat Bran *(Natures Warehouse)*	1		

1 = High Fat	2 = High Sodium	3 = High Refined Sugar	5 = Cholesterol
1+ = Very High Fat	2+ = Very High Sodium	4 = Highly Processed	★= Better Choice

CRACKERS

Crackers are a lot like our breads. There are many of them on the shelf, but only a few can get into *The Food Bible*. Most all the highly processed varieties, such as the popular saltines, are processed with cottonseed oil which cannot be recommended. For example: *Keebler* Zesta Wheat Saltines contain cottonseed oil and artificial color. However, there are some very fine selections from among the better quality whole grain varieties. I feel that we'll be seeing more and more of these good kinds showing up in our stores in the future.

As with other grain products, I try to choose those that will give me the most nutrients per calorie while at the same time will not give me extra high fat and salt.

VARIETY *(Brand)*   RATING CODE

	1	2		4
CRACKERS				
American Classic, Cracked Wheat *(Nabisco)*	1	2		4
American Classic, Golden Sesame *(Nabisco)*	1	2		4
Armenian Thin Bread *(Venus)*		2		4
Better Cheddars *(Nabisco)*	1+	2		4
Better Cheddars, Low Salt *(Nabisco)*	1+			4
Bran Wafers, Salt Free *(Venus)*				4
Brown Rice Snaps, Buckwheat, No Salt *(Edward & Sons)*	★			
Brown Rice Snaps, Buckwheat Tamari *(Edward & Sons)*	★			
Brown Rice Snaps, Onion Garlic *(Edward & Sons)*	★			
Brown Rice Snaps, Parmesan *(Edward & Sons)*	★			
Brown Rice Snaps, Sesame, No Salt *(Edward & Sons)*	★			
Brown Rice Snaps, Tamari Seaweed *(Edward & Sons)*	★			
Brown Rice Snaps, Tamari Sesame *(Edward & Sons)*	★			
Brown Rice Thins, Low Sodium *(Hol.Grain)*	★			
Brown Rice Thins, Sodium Free *(Hol.Grain)*	★			
Cheese *(Hain)*	1			
Cracked Wheat *(Golden Harvest)*	1			4
Cracked Wheat Wafers, Salt Free *(Venus)*				4
Crispbread, Breakfast *(Wasa)*	★			
Crispbread, Fiber Plus *(Wasa)*		2		
Crispbread, Hearty Rye *(Wasa)*		2		
Crispbread, Light Rye *(Finn Crisp)*		2		
Crispbread, Light Rye *(Wasa)*	★			
Crispbread, Rye *(Finn Crisp)*		2		
Crispbread, Rye-Bran *(Kavli)*	★			
Crispbread, Sesame *(Wasa)*	★			
Crispbread, Thick *(Kavli)*	★			
Crispbread, Thin *(Kavli)*	★			
Graham Bites, Brown Sugar 'n Spice *(Nabisco)*			3	4
Graham Bites, Honey 'n Oat Bran *(Nabisco)*			3	4
Harvest Crisps, 5-Grain *(Nabisco)*		2		4
Harvest Crisps, Oat *(Nabisco)*		2		4
Herb Stoned Wheat *(Health Valley)*	1			

1 = High Fat	3 = High Refined Sugar	5 = Cholesterol
1+ = Very High Fat	4 = Highly Processed	★= Better Choice
2 = High Sodium		
2+ = Very High Sodium		

VARIETY (Brand)   RATING CODE

VARIETY (Brand)	★	1	2	4
Herb Stoned Wheat, No Salt *(Health Valley)*		1		
Lavosh *(Golden Harvest)*				4
Light Rye *(RYVTA)*	★			
Matzo Thins, Dietetic *(Manischewitz)*				4
Matzo, Whole Wheat *(Manischewitz)*	★			
Melba Rounds, Garlic *(Devonsheer)*			2	4
Melba Rounds, Oat Bran *(Devonsheer)*			2	4
Melba Rounds, Onion *(Devonsheer)*			2	4
Melba Rounds, Plain *(Devonsheer)*			2	4
Melba Rounds, Rye *(Devonsheer)*			2	4
Melba Rounds, Sesame *(Devonsheer)*			2	4
Melba Rounds, Unsalted Plain *(Devonsheer)*				4
Melba Toast, Honey Bran *(Devonsheer)*			2	4
Melba Toast, Oat Bran *(Devonsheer)*			2	4
Melba Toast, Sesame *(Devonsheer)*			2	4
Melba Toast, Unsalted Wheat *(Devonsheer)*				4
Melba Toast, Wheat *(Devonsheer)*			2	4
Oat Bran Wafers *(Venus)*			2	4
Oat Bran Wafers, Salt Free *(Venus)*				4
Oat Thins *(Nabisco)*		1		4
Onion *(Hain)*		1		
Onion, No Salt *(Hain)*		1		
Rice Bran *(Health Valley)*	★			
Rich Whole Wheat *(Hain)*		1		
Rich Whole Wheat, No Salt *(Hain)*		1		
Ritz Bits *(Nabisco)*		1+	2	4
Ritz Bits, Cheese *(Nabisco)*		1+	2	4
Ritz Bits, Low Salt *(Nabisco)*		1+		4
Rye *(Hain)*			2	
Rye *(Pritikin)*			2	
Rye Wafer *(Venus)*			2	
Rye, No Salt *(Hain)*	★			
Saltines, Whole Wheat Premium Plus *(Nabisco)*			2	4

1 = High Fat   2 = High Sodium   3 = High Refined Sugar   5 = Cholesterol
1+ = Very High Fat   2+ = Very High Sodium   4 = Highly Processed   ★= Better Choice

VARIETY *(Brand)*   RATING CODE

Variety (Brand)	★	1	2	3	4
Sea Toasts *(Keebler)*			2		4
Sesame *(Ak-Mak)*	★				
Sesame *(Hain)*		1	2+		
Sesame Rye *(RYVTA)*	★				
Sesame Stoned Wheat *(Health Valley)*		1			
Sesame Stoned Wheat, No Salt *(Health Valley)*		1			
Sesame Wafers *(Venus)*			2		
Sesame, No Salt *(Hain)*		1			
Sour Cream & Chive *(Hain)*		1			
Sour Cream & Chive, No Salt *(Hain)*		1			
Sourdough *(Hain)*		1	2		
Sourdough, Low Salt *(Hain)*		1			
Stoned Wheat *(Health Valley)*		1			
Stoned Wheat Wafers *(Venus)*			2		4
Stoned Wheat, No Salt *(Health Valley)*		1			
Teddy Grahams, Cinnamon *(Nabisco)*				3	4
Teddy Grahams, Honey *(Nabisco)*				3	4
Teddy Grahams, Vanilla *(Nabisco)*				3	4
Vegetable *(Hain)*		1			
Vegetable, No Salt *(Hain)*		1			
Vegetable, Seven Grain, Stoned Wheat *(Health Valley)*		1			
Vegetable, Seven Grain, Stoned Wheat, No Salt *(Health Valley)*		1			
Waverly *(Nabisco)*		1	2		4
Waverly, Low Salt *(Nabisco)*		1			4
Wheat Thins, Low Salt *(Nabisco)*		1			
Wheat Thins, Nutty *(Nabisco)*		1+	2		
Wheat Thins, Original *(Nabisco)*		1	2		
Wheatines, Lightly Salted Tops *(Barbara's)*			2		
Wheatines, Unsalted Tops *(Barbara's)*	★				
Wheatsworth *(Nabisco)*		1	2		4
Whole Wheat Thins, Low Sodium *(Hol.Grain)*	★				
Whole Wheat Thins, Sodium Free *(Hol.Grain)*	★				

1 = High Fat 2 = High Sodium 3 = High Refined Sugar 5 = Cholesterol
1+ = Very High Fat 2+ = Very High Sodium 4 = Highly Processed ★= Better Choice

DESSERTS

The puddings, gelatins, custards, and mousses — as well as most other desserts — didn't make *The Food Bible*. The items I have included I don't really consider to be food. When we eat something that is high in fat, high in sodium, very highly processed, and with egg yolks added to increase the cholesterol, we're asking for big trouble if we make a habit of eating these "foods." You'll find some better choices for desserts and sweet-type items under Snacks.

I rarely purchase a prepared dessert, but if I do, a fruit pie would be my choice. When I make a gelatin dessert, I use *Knox* unflavored gelatin and fruit juices, then add my own fruit. By doing this, I eliminate the additives and preservatives in most all fruit-flavored gelatins such as *Jell-O*.

VARIETY *(Brand)*   RATING CODE

DESSERTS
FROZEN

Apple Cobbler *(Marie Callender's)*	1	3	
Apple'n Spice Bake Dessert Light *(Pepperidge Farm)*		3	
Berry Cobbler *(Marie Callender's)*	1	3	
Brownie Cheesecake *(Lindy's)*	1+	3	5
Cheese Cake *(Lindy's)*	1+	3	5
Cheesecake, Strawberry *(Pepperidge Farm)*	1+	3	5
Cherry Cobbler *(Marie Callender's)*	1	3	
Cinnamon Rolls *(Sara Lee)*	1+	3	4
Coffee Cake, Apple Cinnamon *(Sara Lee)*	1+	3	4
Coffee Cake, Butter Pecan *(Sara Lee)*	1+	3	4
Coffee Cake, Butter Streusel *(Sara Lee)*	1+	3	4
Coffee Cake, Cheese *(Sara Lee)*	1	3	4
Fudge Cakes, Individual *(Sara Lee)*	1+	3	4	5
Peach Cobbler *(Marie Callender's)*	1	3	
Pie Crust *(Mrs. Smith's)*	1+		4
Pound Cake, Butter *(Sara Lee)*	1+	3	4
Pound Cakes, Individual *(Sara Lee)*	1+	3	4	5
Puff Pastry Shells *(Pepperidge Farm)*	1+		4
Sweet Roll, Apple *(Weight Watchers)*		3	4

PACKAGED

Gelatin, *(Unflavored Knox)*	★
Tapioca Pearls *(Gourmet Award)*	★
Tapioca Pearls *(Reese)*	★

---

1 = High Fat   2 = High Sodium   3 = High Refined Sugar   5 = Cholesterol
1+ = Very High Fat   2+ = Very High Sodium   4 = Highly Processed   ★= Better Choice

DIET FOODS

In my opinion, many diet food products are not healthful. Most dessert-type products contain NutraSweet or saccharin, and many low-salt products are very high in potassium which can lead to health problems. I prefer using natural fruit juices as sweeteners and lowering sodium without increasing potassium. Also, many diet foods use additives to make them taste better. Remember that all fresh and most frozen fruits and vegetables do not have sweeteners, sodium, additives or preservatives added to them, making them much better choices.

VARIETY *(Brand)*   RATING CODE

DIET FOODS			
Applesauce *(Featherweight)*	★		
Applesauce *(Nutradiet)*	★		
Apricots *(Featherweight)*	★		
Apricots *(Nutradiet)*	★		
Baking Powder, Low Sodium *(Featherweight)*	★		
Butter Buds *(Butter Buds)*		2+ 3	4
Carrots, Sliced *(Nutradiet)*	★		
Catsup *(Featherweight)*	★		
Catsup *(Weight Watchers)*		2+ 3	
Corn *(Featherweight)*	★		
Corn, Cream Style *(Nutradiet)*	★		
Corn, Whole Kernel *(Nutradiet)*	★		
Crispbread, Garlic *(Weight Watchers)*		2	4
Crispbread, Golden Wheat *(Weight Watchers)*		2	4
Crispbread, Harvest Rice *(Weight Watchers)*		2	4
Dairy Creamer *(Weight Watchers)*	★		
Grapefruit Sections *(Featherweight)*	★		
Grapefruit Sections *(Nutradiet)*	★		
Green Beans *(Featherweight)*	★		
Green Beans *(Nutradiet)*	★		
Mixed Vegetables *(Featherweight)*	★		
Molly McButter, Butter Flavor *(Molly McButter)*		2+ 3	4
Molly McButter, Cheese Flavor *(Molly McButter)*		2+ 3	4
Molly McButter, Sour Cream Flavor *(Molly McButter)*		2+ 3	4
Munchies, Chocolate Fudge *(Skinny Haven)*		3	
Munchies, Nacho Cheese *(Skinny Haven)*	1	2	
Munchies, Toasted Onion *(Skinny Haven)*	1	2	
Peach Slices, Lite Fruits *(Featherweight)*	★		
Peaches *(Featherweight)*	★		
Peaches *(Nutradiet)*	★		
Pears *(Featherweight)*	★		
Pears *(Nutradiet)*	★		
Peas *(Featherweight)*	★		

1 = High Fat	2 = High Sodium	3 = High Refined Sugar	5 = Cholesterol
1+ = Very High Fat	2+ = Very High Sodium	4 = Highly Processed	★= Better Choice

VARIETY *(Brand)*   RATING CODE

Peas & Carrots *(Nutradiet)*	★			
Pickles, Sliced *(Featherweight)*	★			
Popcorn, Microwave *(Weight Watchers)*	★			
Salmon, Pink, No Salt Added *(Featherweight)*	1			5
Spaghetti Sauce, Meat-Flavored *(Weight Watchers)*		2+		
Spaghetti Sauce, Mushroom *(Weight Watchers)*		2+		
Spinach *(Featherweight)*	★			
Tomatoes *(Nutradiet)*	★			
Tuna, Chunk Light, No Salt Added *(Featherweight)*				5

DINNERS, ENTRÉES AND SIDE DISHES

Our demand for convenience foods has given the manufacturers a play house. Buy one of these, whip it in the microwave and presto — an instant meal. Many dinners of this type contain additives and preservatives; thus, they're eliminated from *The Food Bible.* As a group, these boxed and canned products are on a par with some restaurant meals where fat, salt and highly processed foods are used quite plentifully. As with restaurant eating, we just need to choose carefully.

Please note: Most of these dinners, entrées, and side dishes are not complete meals. They are heavy on the protein (meats and cheeses), use processed pastas, and offer very few vegetables. By adding whole wheat bread, a potato and some raw or lightly cooked veggies, you can "up" the quality of these products tremendously.

I am very quick-and-easy conscious, so I like the convenience of these dinners, entrées and side dishes, but I try to be real choosy; then add a little health back into them when I get home. With all the ratings, you probably think I put the worst ones in *The Food Bible,* but unfortunately these are the best offered. However, I think we'll be seeing some better boxed and canned choices in the future.

Normally, I would think that frozen dinners would not have the additives and preservatives that their non-frozen counterparts have. But we frequently find them in these products — particularly the flavor enhancers. You see, processing destroys flavor, so it is added back in an artificial form. Let's look at a couple examples and see the additives and preservatives that are used.

Stouffer's Lean Cuisine Cheese Cannelloni	MSG, BHA & BHT
Weight Watchers Stuffed Sole with Newburg Sauce	cottonseed oil, artificial flavor, MSG, disodium guanylate & disodium inosinate

Do you see why so many didn't make *The Food Bible*? As a group, these rate about like the boxed and canned.

VARIETY (Brand)   RATING CODE

DINNERS, ENTRÉES, AND SIDE DISHES
BOXED AND CANNED

Product	★	Fat	Sodium	Processed	Cholesterol
ABC's & 123's, Spaghetti Sauce with Cheese (Chef Boyardee)			2+	4	
Amaranth with Vegetables, Fast Menu (Health Valley)	★				
Beef Stew, Hearty Family Favorites (Lipton)			2		
Black Bean with Vegetables, Fast Menu (Health Valley)	★				
Brown & Wild Rice, Mushroom Recipe (Uncle Ben's)			2+	4	
Brown Rice, Quick Vegetable & Herb (Arrowhead Mills)	★				
Brown Rice, Quick Wild Rice & Herbs (Arrowhead Mills)			2		
Burger Mix, Nature's, Original (Fantastic Foods)	★				
Burger Mix, Nature's, Pizza (Fantastic Foods)			2+		
Cheese Tortellini, Impromptu (Kraft)			2+	4	5
Chicken Cacciatori, Impromptu Lite (Kraft)			2+	4	5
Chicken Oriental, Minute Gourmet (Hunt's)			2+	4	
Chicken, Meatless Style (Hain)			2+		
Chili Fixin's, Manwich (Hunt's)			2+		
Chili Mix, Vegetarian with Beans (Fantastic Foods)			2		
Chili with Beans (Gebhardt)		1+	2+		5
Chili with Beans (Wolf)		1+	2+		5
Chili with Chicken (Hain)			2+		5
Chili without Beans (Gebhardt)		1+	2		5
Chili without Beans (Wolf)		1+	2		5
Chili, Chicken, Low Sodium (Shelton's)	★				
Chili, Chicken, Mild (Shelton's)			2+		
Chili, Chicken, Spicy (Shelton's)			2+		
Chili, Hot with Beans (Hormel)		1+	2+		5
Chili, Jalapeño with Beans (Wolf)		1+	2+		5
Chili, Jalapeño without Beans (Wolf)		1+	2		5
Chili, Mild Vegetarian with Beans (Health Valley)			2+		
Chili, Mild Vegetarian with Beans, No Salt (Health Valley)	★				
Chili, Mild Vegetarian with Lentils (Health Valley)			2		
Chili, Mild Vegetarian with Lentils, No Salt (Health Valley)	★				
Chili, Spicy Vegetarian (Health Valley)			2+		
Chili, Spicy Vegetarian, No Salt (Health Valley)	★				
Chili, Turkey, Low Sodium (Shelton's)	★				

1 = High Fat   2 = High Sodium   3 = High Refined Sugar   5 = Cholesterol
1+ = Very High Fat   2+ = Very High Sodium   4 = Highly Processed   ★= Better Choice

VARIETY *(Brand)*   RATING CODE

VARIETY (Brand)	★	1	2	2+	3	4	5
Chili, Turkey, Mild *(Shelton's)*				2+			
Chili, Turkey, Spicy *(Shelton's)*				2+			
Chow Mein, Mandarin, Prepared, No Butter *(Fantastic Foods)*		1		2+			
Circus O's, Plain *(Franco American)*				2+		4	
Circus O's, with Meatballs *(Franco American)*				2+		4	
Dinosaurs, Cheese *(Chef Boyardee)*				2+		4	
Fettucini, Marinara *(Lunch Bucket)*				2+		4	
Hamburger Italiano, Hearty Lasagna, Prepared *(Chef Boyardee)*		1		2+	3	4	5
Hamburger Italiano, Pizza Spirals, Prepared *(Chef Boyardee)*		1		2+	3	4	5
Hamburger Italiano, Zesty Twists, Prepared *(Chef Boyardee)*		1		2+	3	4	5
Hearty Soup, Country Vegetable Micro Cup *(Hormel)*				2+			
Herb Side Dish *(Hain)*				2+			
Kid's Kitchen Spaghetti Rings *(Hormel)*				2+		4	
Lasagna *(Lunch Bucket)*				2+		4	
Lasagna, Garden Vegetable Sauce *(Chef Boyardee)*				2+		4	
Lentil with Vegetables, Fast Menu *(Health Valley)*	★						
Long Grain & Wild Rice, Original Recipe *(Uncle Ben's)*				2+		4	
Long Grain & Wild Rice, Original Fast Cooking *(Uncle Ben's)*				2+		4	
Macaroni & Cheese, Artichoke *(DeBoles)*						4	
Macaroni & Cheese, Whole Wheat *(DeBoles)*	★						
Macaroni & Cheese, Whole Wheat *(Hodgson Mill)*	★						
Macaroni & Cheese, Whole Wheat with Cheddar *(Fantastic Foods)*			2				
Macaroni & Cheese, Whole Wheat with Parmesan Herb, Prepared *(Fantastic Foods)*			2				
Macaroni 'n Beef *(Lunch Bucket)*				2+		4	
Manicotti, Impromptu *(Kraft)*		1	2			4	
Noodle & Cheese, Artichoke *(DeBoles)*						4	
Noodles & Sauce, Butter *(Lipton)*				2+		4	
Noodles & Sauce, Butter & Herb *(Lipton)*				2+		4	
Noodles & Sauce, Parmesan *(Lipton)*				2+		4	
Noodles & Sauce, Sour Cream & Chive *(Lipton)*				2+		4	
Not-So-Sloppy Joe *(Hormel)*				2+	3		
Oat Bran Fettucini, Herb Italiano *(Health Valley)*	★						
Oat Bran Fettucini, Marinara *(Health Valley)*	★						

1 = High Fat   2 = High Sodium   3 = High Refined Sugar   5 = Cholesterol
1+ = Very High Fat   2+ = Very High Sodium   4 = Highly Processed   ★ = Better Choice

VARIETY (Brand) RATING CODE

Item (Brand)	★	Code	Code
Oat Bran Fettucini, Primavera (Health Valley)	★		
Oat Bran Pilaf with Vegetables, Fast Menu (Health Valley)		2	
Pac-Man, Cheese Flavor (Chef Boyardee)		2+	4
Pasta & Cheddar Cheese (Minute)		2+	4
Pasta & Sauce, Creamy Parmesan (Hain)		2	
Pasta & Sauce, Creamy Swiss (Hain)		2	
Pasta & Sauce, Fettuccine Alfredo (Hain)		2	
Pasta & Sauce, Italian Herb (Hain)	★		
Pasta & Sauce, Marinara (Hain)		2+	
Pasta & Sauce, Primavera (Hain)		2+	
Pasta & Sauce, Tangy Cheddar (Hain)		2	
Pasta Salad, Italian Herb, Prepared (Fantastic Foods)	1		
Pasta Salad, Spicy Oriental, Prepared (Fantastic Foods)	1+		
Pasta, Four Cheese (Ronzoni)		2+	4
Pasta, Italiano (Lunch Bucket)		2+	4
Pilaf, Barley (Near East)		2+	
Pilaf, Lentil (Near East)		2+	4
Pilaf, Rice (Vigo)		2+	4
Pilaf Mix, Brown Rice (Near East)		2+	
Pilaf Mix, Brown Rice with Miso (Fantastic Foods)		2	
Pilaf Mix, Curry Rice (Near East)		2+	4
Pilaf Mix, Rice (Near East)		2+	4
Pilaf Mix, Savory Couscous (Fantastic Foods)		2	
Pilaf Mix, Spanish Brown Rice (Fantastic Foods)		2+	
Pilaf Mix, Three Grain with Herbs (Fantastic Foods)		2	
Pilaf Mix, Wheat (Near East)		2+	4
Polenta (Fantastic Foods)		2	
Potatoes au Gratin, Prepared, No Butter (Fantastic Foods)		2	
Potatoes Country Style, Prepared, No Butter (Fantastic Foods)		2+	
Potatoes, Mashed (Barbara's)	★		
Potatoes, Mashed, Unpeeled (Barbara's)	★		
RavioliOs, Beef (Franco American)		2+	4
Rice & Sauce, Cajun Style (Lipton)		2+	4

1 = High Fat 2 = High Sodium 3 = High Refined Sugar 5 = Cholesterol
1+ = Very High Fat 2+ = Very High Sodium 4 = Highly Processed ★ = Better Choice

VARIETY *(Brand)* — RATING CODE

Food (Brand)	1	1+	2	2+	3	4	5	★
Rice Almondine *(Hain)*	1		2					
Rice Oriental, 3-Grain Goodness *(Hain)*	1		2					
Shells & Cheddar, Artichoke *(DeBoles)*						4		
Shells in Tomato Sauce with Mushrooms *(Chef Boyardee)*				2+		4		
Shells 'n Curry, Tofu Classic, Prepared, No Butter *(Fantastic Foods)*			2					
Smurf, Cheese *(Franco American)*				2+		4		
Spaghetti 'n Meat Sauce *(Lunch Bucket)*				2+		4		
Spaghetti Dinner with Meat Sauce *(Chef Boyardee)*			2			4		
Spaghetti in Tomato Sauce with Cheese *(Franco American)*				2+		4		
Spaghetti with Meatballs *(Franco American)*	1			2+		4		
SpaghettiOs with Meat Balls *(Franco American)*	1			2+		4		
SpaghettiOs, Tomato & Cheese *(Franco American)*				2+		4		
Spanish Brown Rice *(Pritikin)*								★
Spanish Rice Mix *(Near East)*				2+		4		
Spanish Rice, Quick Cooking *(Arrowhead Mills)*			2					
Sporty O's in Tomato & Cheese Sauce *(Franco American)*				2+		4		
Sporty O's, Meatballs *(Franco American)*	1			2+		4		
Stroganoff, Tofu Classic, Prepared, No Butter *(Fantastic Foods)*			2					
Sweet & Sour Chicken Mix, Minute Gourmet *(Hunt's)*			2		3			
Tabouli, Prepared *(Fantastic Foods)*		1+	2					
Tamales in Chili Gravy *(Wolf)*		1+		2+			5	
Teddy O's in Tomato & Cheese Sauce *(Franco American)*				2+		4		
Teddy O's, Meatballs *(Franco American)*	1			2+		4		
Tic Tac Toes, Cheese Sauce *(Chef Boyardee)*				2+		4		
Tofu Burger, Prepared *(Fantastic Foods)*	1		2					
Tofu Scrambler Mix, Prepared, No Butter *(Fantastic Foods)*	1		2					
Tortellini, Cheese *(DaVinci)*			2			4		
Tortellini, Cheese *(Vigo)*			2			4	5	
Tortellini, Cheese, Tomato, Egg & Spinach *(Vigo)*			2			4	5	
Tortellini, Multi-Color with Cheese *(DaVinci)*			2			4		
Tortellini, Ravioletti with Cheese *(DaVinci)*			2			4		
Tortellini, Spinach with Cheese *(DaVinci)*			2			4		
Twists in Pizza Sauce *(Franco American)*				2+		4		

1 = High Fat 1+ = Very High Fat 2 = High Sodium 2+ = Very High Sodium 3 = High Refined Sugar 4 = Highly Processed 5 = Cholesterol ★ = Better Choice

VARIETY (Brand)

RATING CODE

Food (Brand)	Fat	Sodium	Sugar	Processed	Cholesterol
Vegetable Lasagna, Impromptu Lite (Kraft)	1	2+		4	
Vegetarian Beans with Miso (Health Valley)	★				

DINNERS, ENTRÉES, SIDE DISHES: FROZEN

Food (Brand)	Fat	Sodium	Sugar	Processed	Cholesterol
Agnolotti, Broccoli & Cheddar (Putney Pasta)	1	2		4	5
Agnolotti, Pesto (Putney Pasta)	1	2		4	5
Broccoli Stuffed Shells (Celentano)	1+	2		4	5
Cannelloni Florentine (Celentano)	1	2		4	5
Cannelloni, Chicken, Light (Le Menu)		2+		4	5
Cashew Chicken (Stouffer's)		2+		4	5
Cheddar Potatoes & Broccoli, Side Dish (Budget Gourmet)	1	2			5
Cheese Enchilada (Kraft)	1+	2		4	5
Cheese Ravioli (Swanson)	1	2+		4	5
Cheese Tortellini, Side Dish (Budget Gourmet)				4	
Chicken & Noodle, Broccoli (Budget Gourmet)	1+	2		4	5
Chicken a la King (Swanson)		2+		4	5
Chicken a la King, Light (Le Menu)		2		4	5
Chicken Breast Fillets, Italian (Tyson)		2+			5
Chicken Chunks, Bugs Bunny Looney Tunes (Tyson)	1	2			
Chicken Enchilada (Van de Kamp's)	1	2+			5
Chicken Parmigiana (Celentano)	1	2		4	5
Chicken Primavera (Celentano)		2		4	5
Cream Style Corn (Green Giant)		2+			
Dumplings (Reames)				4	5
Egg Noodles (Reames)				4	5
Egg Rolls, Chicken (Lana's)		2			
Egg Rolls, Pork (Lana's)		2			
Egg Rolls, Shrimp (Lana's)		2			
Egg Rolls, Vegetable (Lana's)		2			
Eggplant Parmigiana (Celentano)	1+			4	5
Eggplant Rollettes (Celentano)	1+			4	5
Enchiladas, Cheese (Café Mexico)	1	2+		4	
Fettucini Alfredo (Kraft)	1+	2		4	5

1 = High Fat
1+ = Very High Fat
2 = High Sodium
2+ = Very High Sodium
3 = High Refined Sugar
4 = Highly Processed
5 = Cholesterol
★= Better Choice

VARIETY *(Brand)* — RATING CODE

	1	2	3	4	5
Garden Vegetables Lasagna, Light *(Le Menu)*		2		4	5
Kid Cuisine, Mini Cheese Ravioli *(Banquet)*		2	3	4	
Lasagna *(Celentano)*	1			4	5
Lasagna *(Weight Watchers)*		2+		4	5
Lasagna Primavera *(Celentano)*		2		4	5
Lasagna with Meat Sauce *(Kraft)*	1	2		4	5
Lasagna with Meat Sauce, Light *(Le Menu)*		2		4	5
Lasagna, Italian Sausage *(Budget Gourmet)*	1	2		4	5
Lasagna, Meat Sauce *(Stouffers)*	1	2		4	5
Lasagna, Three Cheese *(Budget Gourmet)*	1	2		4	5
Lasagna, Zucchini, Lean Cuisine *(Stouffers)*		2+		4	5
Macaroni & Beef *(Swanson)*		2+		4	5
Macaroni & Beef in Sauce *(Kraft)*	1	2+		4	5
Macaroni & Cheese, One Serving *(Green Giant)*	1	2		4	
Macaroni & Cheese, Side Dish *(Budget Gourmet)*	1+	2		4	5
Macaroni & Cheese, Tweedy Looney Tunes *(Tyson)*		2		4	
Manicotti *(Celentano)*	1	2		4	5
Manicotti, Cheese *(Domani)*	1	2		4	5
Manicotti, Cheese *(John's)*	1	2		4	5
Manicotti, Cheese *(Weight Watchers)*	1	2		4	5
Manicotti, Cheese, Meat Sauce *(Budget Gourmet)*	1+	2		4	5
Meat Sauce & Cheese Tortellini, Light *(Le Menu)*		2		4	
New England Vegetables, Side Dish *(Budget Gourmet)*	1+	2			5
Oriental Rice with Vegetables, Side Dish *(Budget Gourmet)*	1	2		4	5
Pasta & Cheese *(Celentano)*	1			4	5
Pasta Accents, Garden Herb *(Green Giant)*	1	2		4	
Pasta in Marinara Sauce, One Serving *(Green Giant)*		2+		4	
Pasta plus Oriental Vegetables *(C & W)*				4	
Pasta plus Petite Vegetables *(C & W)*				4	
Pasta, Sweet Peas & Cheese, One Serving *(Green Giant)*		2+		4	
Peas & Pearl Onions, Classic Mixture *(Birds Eye)*		2+			
Pilaf, Asparagus, Garden Gourmet *(Green Giant)*		2+		4	
Pizza, Cheese *(McCain)*	1	2		4	5

1 = High Fat   2 = High Sodium   3 = High Refined Sugar   5 = Cholesterol
1+ = Very High Fat   2+ = Very High Sodium   4 = Highly Processed   ★= Better Choice

VARIETY (Brand) — RATING CODE

Item	1	2	4	5
Pizza, Cheese Turtles (McCain Ellio's)	1	2	4	5
Pizza, Deluxe Combination (Weight Watchers)		2	4	5
Pizza, Double Cheese (Tony's)	1	2	4	5
Pizza, Extra Cheese Turtles (McCain Ellio's)	1	2+	4	5
Pizza, Four Cheese (Wolfgang-Puck's)	1+	2+	4	5
Pizza, Lite (Old Chicago)	★			
Pizza, Pizsoy (Tree Tavern)	★			
Pizza, Sausage & Herbs (Wolfgang-Puck's)	1	2	4	5
Pizza, Spicy Chicken (Wolfgang-Puck's)	1	2	4	5
Ravioli, Baked Cheese (Weight Watchers)	1	2	4	5
Ravioli, Beef (Domani)	1	2	4	5
Ravioli, Beef (Mamma Lina's)	1	2	4	5
Ravioli, Cheese (Domani)	1	2	4	5
Ravioli, Cheese (John's)	1	2	4	5
Ravioli, Cheese (Mamma Lina's)	1	2	4	5
Ravioli, Cheese Light (Budget Gourmet)	1	2+	4	5
Ravioli, Jumbo Cheese (John's)	1	2	4	5
Ravioli, Meat (John's)	1	2	4	5
Ravioli, Mini (Celentano)			4	5
Raviolini, Cheddar & Walnuts (Putney Pasta)	1	2	4	5
Rice Mexicana, Side Dish (Budget Gourmet)			4	
Rice Pilaf with Green Beans, Side Dish (Budget Gourmet)	1	2	4	5
Rotini Cheddar, Garden Gourmet (Green Giant)	1	2	4	
Sherry Wild Rice, Garden Gourmet (Green Giant)		2	4	
Shrimp Gumbo (Stilwell)		2+		5
Sirloin Chili Size with Steak Fries (Kraft)	1+	2		5
Sirloin Enchilada, Ranchero, Light (Budget Gourmet)	1	2		
Sirloin of Beef, Herb Sauce, Light (Budget Gourmet)	1	2	4	5
Sirloin Tips with Noodles in Burgundy (Budget Gourmet)	1	2	4	5
Sirloin Tips with Noodles (Swanson)	1	2	4	
Spaghetti & Italian Style Meatballs (Swanson)	1	2	4	5
Spaghetti with Beef Sauce, Light (Le Menu)		2	4	
Spaghetti with Meat Sauce (Kraft)	1	2	4	5

1 = High Fat   2 = High Sodium   3 = High Refined Sugar   5 = Cholesterol
1+ = Very High Fat   2+ = Very High Sodium   4 = Highly Processed   ★ = Better Choice

VARIETY *(Brand)*   RATING CODE

VARIETY (Brand)	1	2	3	4	5
Spring Vegetables in Cheese Sauce, Side Dish *(Budget Gourmet)*	1+	2			5
Stuffed Shells *(Celentano)*		2		4	5
Stuffed Shells *(Domani)*	1	2		4	5
Stuffed Shells, Cheese *(John's)*	1	2		4	5
Sweet & Sour Chicken *(Kibun Gold)*			3	4	5
Tamales, Blue Corn with Chicken *(Col. Sanchez)*	1				5
Tamales, Green Chili with Cheese *(Col. Sanchez)*	1+				5
Tamales, Red Chili with Tofu *(Col. Sanchez)*	1+	2			
Teriyaki Chicken Breast, Light & Lively *(Budget Gourmet)*				4	5
Tortellini, Cheese *(Weight Watchers)*		2		4	
Tortellini, Meat Sauce & Cheese, Light *(Le Menu)*		2			
Tortellini, Provencal, Garden Gourmet *(Green Giant)*		2+		4	
Turkey Swiss Turnovers, Oven Stuff *(Quaker)*	1	2			5
Turkey, Glazed with Rice & Vegetables, Light *(Le Menu)*		2		4	5
Veal Parmigiana & Spaghetti *(Swanson)*	1	2+		4	5
Vegetables with Creamy Mushroom Sauce *(Birds Eye)*		2+			
Vegetarian Medley *(Kibun Gold)*	★				
White Corn in Butter Sauce *(Green Giant)*		2			
DINNERS, ENTRÉES, SIDE DISHES: REFRIGERATED					
Agnolotti with Basil & Cheese *(Contadina)*				4	5
Chicken By George, Cajun Style *(Hormel)*	1	2			5
Chicken By George, Country Mustard & Dill *(Hormel)*	1	2			5
Chicken By George, Italian Blue Cheese *(Hormel)*	1	2+			5
Chicken By George, Lemon Herb *(Hormel)*		2+			5
Chicken By George, Mexican Style *(Hormel)*	1	2			5
Chicken By George, Teriyaki *(Hormel)*		2			5
Chicken By George, Tomato Herb *(Hormel)*	1	2			5
Ravioli with Cheese *(Contadina)*		2		4	5
Ravioli with Cheese *(Romance)*		2		4	5
Ravioli with Meat *(Contadina)*				4	5
Ravioli with Meat *(Romance)*		2		4	5
Spinach Tortellini with Cheese *(Contadina)*		2		4	5
Tortellini with Cheese *(Contadina)*		2		4	5
Tortellini with Cheese *(Romance)*		2		4	5

1 = High Fat   2 = High Sodium   3 = High Refined Sugar   5 = Cholesterol
1+ = Very High Fat   2+ = Very High Sodium   4 = Highly Processed   ★= Better Choice

VARIETY *(Brand)*   **RATING CODE**

Tortellini with Meat *(Contadina)*	2	4	5
Tortellini with Meat *(Romance)*	2	4	5
Tortelloni with Spinach *(Romance)*	2	4	5
Turkey By George, Italian Style Parmesan *(Hormel)*	1 2+		5
Turkey By George, Lemon Pepper *(Hormel)*	2+		5
Turkey By George, Mustard Tarragon *(Hormel)*	1 2+		5

1 = High Fat	2 = High Sodium	3 = High Refined Sugar	5 = Cholesterol
1+ = Very High Fat	2+ = Very High Sodium	4 = Highly Processed	★= Better Choice

FRUITS

Fruits are offered fresh, frozen, dried and canned, and most are free of additives and preservatives. The question I most often hear is, "Which are the best?" Some choices may be personal, but I rate fruits pretty much this way: I will always choose *fresh fruits* first if they are grown locally and picked ripe or very close to ripe.

However, if I'm in Chicago and see "fresh" fruits from California on the shelves, I may rate them last. First of all, they're picked green and will generally be tasteless. But the biggest risk I see is the chemicals they're subjected to while in transit. Many times truckers are required to spray gases to speed up ripening or slow it down, and if bugs appear, they must spray chemicals to kill the bugs. Somehow I feel that the concept of "fresh" is lost in this process.

Canned fruits, in my opinion, do not rate quite as high nutritionally as frozen. The heating process of canning will destroy some vitamins, especially vitamin C. But on the positive side, canned fruits, those packed in water, can still be nutritious, and we have good selections from which to choose.

Dried fruits are very nutritious; however, they may contain the preservatives known as sulfites. Sulfites are antioxidants and are used to keep foods from turning dark. They are most prevalent on light-colored fruits such as apricots, peaches, apples and so on.

Frozen fruits will usually be more uniform in quality as they are generally harvested and processed in the same area. They are picked closer to the ripe stage and are not subjected to cross-country rides. I really like our frozen fruit selections, especially the ones without sugar added. In addition to the national brands listed in *The Food Bible*, you will find some excellent local brands.

VARIETY *(Brand)*   RATING CODE

FRUITS
CANNED

Variety (Brand)	Better Choice	Rating
Apple Slices, Homestyle *(Musselman's)*		3
Apple, Peach, Fruit Classics *(Gerber)*		3
Apple, Raspberry, Fruit Classics *(Gerber)*		3
Apples, Sliced *(Musselman's)*	★	
Apples, Sliced *(Thank You)*	★	
Applesauce *(Lucky Leaf)*		3
Applesauce *(Mott's)*		3
Applesauce *(Musselman's)*		3
Applesauce *(New Morning)*	★	
Applesauce *(Rainbow)*		3
Applesauce *(S & W)*		3
Applesauce *(Seneca)*		3
Applesauce *(Stokely's)*		3
Applesauce *(Town House)*		3
Applesauce *(White House)*		3
Applesauce, 100% Natural *(Seneca)*	★	
Applesauce, Chunky *(Mott's)*		3
Applesauce, Chunky *(Musselman's)*		3
Applesauce, Chunky *(ReNa)*		3
Applesauce, Chunky *(White House)*		3
Applesauce, Cinnamon *(Mott's)*		3
Applesauce, Cinnamon *(Musselman's)*		3
Applesauce, Cinnamon *(Tree Top)*		3
Applesauce, Cinnamon, Fruit Classics *(Gerber)*		3
Applesauce, Dutch Apple Spice *(Mott's)*		3
Applesauce, Fruit Classics *(Gerber)*		3
Applesauce, Granny Smith *(Musselman's)*		3
Applesauce, Natural *(Mott's)*	★	
Applesauce, Natural *(Musselman's)*	★	
Applesauce, Natural *(Tree Top)*	★	
Applesauce, Natural Plus *(White House)*	★	
Applesauce, Natural, Cinnamon *(Musselman's)*	★	
Applesauce, Natural, Fruit Classics *(Gerber)*	★	

VARIETY *(Brand)*   RATING CODE

	Rating
Applesauce, No Sugar *(Country Pure)*	★
Applesauce, Original *(Apple Time)*	★
Applesauce, Original *(Tree Top)*	3
Applesauce, Sodium Free *(Musselman's)*	3
Applesauce, Unsweetened *(S & W)*	★
Apricot Halves *(Del Monte)*	3
Apricot Halves *(Gourmet Award)*	★
Apricot Halves *(Town House)*	3
Apricot Halves, [Lift Top Can] *(Town House)*	3
Apricot Halves, Lite *(Libby's)*	★
Apricots, Lite *(Del Monte)*	3
Apricots, Peeled *(S & W)*	3
Blackberries *(Oregon)*	3
Blackberries *(S & W)*	3
Blackberries *(Thank You)*	3
Blueberries *(Musselman's)*	3
Blueberries *(Oregon)*	3
Blueberries *(S & W)*	3
Blueberries *(Thank You)*	3
Boysenberries *(Oregon)*	3
Boysenberries *(Thank You)*	3
Cherries *(Stokely's)*	★
Cherries, Bing, Dark *(Oregon)*	3
Cherries, Dark *(Oregon)*	3
Cherries, Dark Sweet *(Del Monte)*	3
Cherries, Dark Sweet *(S & W)*	3
Cherries, Dark Sweet *(Thank You)*	3
Cherries, Light Sweet *(S & W)*	3
Cherries, Red Tart *(Musselman's)*	★
Cherries, Royal Anne *(Thank You)*	3
Cherries, Royal Anne, Light *(Oregon)*	3
Cherries, Tart Red *(Thank You)*	★
Cranberry Sauce, Jellied *(Ocean Spray)*	3

1 = High Fat	2 = High Sodium	3 = High Refined Sugar	5 = Cholesterol
1+ = Very High Fat	2+ = Very High Sodium	4 = Highly Processed	★= Better Choice

VARIETY *(Brand)*   RATING CODE

Cranberry Sauce, Whole Berry *(Ocean Spray)*	3
CranFruit-Cranberry, Applesauce *(Ocean Spray)*	3
CranFruit-Cranberry, Orange Sauce *(Ocean Spray)*	3
CranFruit-Cranberry, Raspberry Sauce *(Ocean Spray)*	3
CranFruit-Cranberry, Strawberry Sauce *(Ocean Spray)*	3
Escalloped Apples *(White House)*	3
Figs, Kadota *(Oregon)*	3
Figs, Kadota, Whole *(S & W)*	3
Figs, Whole *(Del Monte)*	3
Fruit Cup, Diced Peaches *(Del Monte)*	3
Fruit Cup, Diced Peaches, Lite *(Del Monte)*	3
Fruit Cup, Mixed Fruit *(Del Monte)*	3
Fruit Cup, Mixed Fruit, Lite *(Del Monte)*	3
Fruit Cup, Pears *(Del Monte)*	3
Fruit Cup, Pineapple *(Del Monte)*	★
Fruit Mix, Light *(Rainbow)*	3
Fruit Naturals, Peaches, Sliced *(Del Monte)*	★
Fruit Naturals, Pear Halves *(Del Monte)*	★
Fruit Pak, Chunky Applesauce & Peach *(Mott's)*	3
Fruit Pak, Chunky Applesauce & Pineapple *(Mott's)*	3
Fruit Salad, Tropical *(Dole)*	3
Grapefruit Sections *(Donald Duck)*	★
Grapefruit Sections *(Gourmet Award)*	★
Grapefruit Sections *(S & W)*	★
Grapefruit Sections *(Stokely's)*	3
Grapefruit Sections *(Town House)*	★
Grapefruit Sections, Light Syrup *(Donald Duck)*	3
Grapefruit Sections, Light Syrup *(Old South)*	3
Grapes, Seedless *(Thank You)*	3
Grapes, Thompson Seedless *(Oregon)*	3
Mandarin Orange Segments *(Dole)*	3
Mandarin Oranges *(Del Monte)*	3
Mandarin Oranges *(Dole)*	3

VARIETY *(Brand)*   RATING CODE

VARIETY (Brand)		RATING CODE
Mandarin Oranges *(Geisha)*		3
Mandarin Oranges *(Gourmet Award)*		3
Mandarin Oranges *(Rainbow)*		3
Mandarin Oranges *(S & W)*	★	
Mandarin Oranges *(3-Diamonds)*		3
Mandarin Oranges *(3-Pearls)*		3
Mandarin Oranges *(Wel-Pac)*		3
Mandarin Oranges, Light Syrup *(Del Monte)*		3
Mango, Sliced *(KA-ME)*		3
Mincemeat *(Borden)*		3
Peach Halves, Lite *(Country Pure)*	★	
Peach Halves, Lite *(Del Monte)*		3
Peach Halves, Lite *(Libby's)*	★	
Peaches *(Argo)*		3
Peaches *(Gardenside)*		3
Peaches, Cling *(Town House)*		3
Peaches, Sliced *(Argo)*		3
Peaches, Sliced & Halves *(Del Monte)*		3
Peaches, Sliced *(S & W)*		3
Peaches, Sliced, Freestone *(Del Monte)*		3
Peaches, Sliced, Lite *(Country Pure)*	★	
Peaches, Sliced, Lite *(Del Monte)*		3
Peaches, Sliced, Lite *(Libby's)*	★	
Peaches, Spiced, Whole *(Del Monte)*		3
Pear Halves *(Del Monte)*		3
Pear Halves, Lite *(Libby's)*	★	
Pears *(Gardenside)*		3
Pears *(S & W)*		3
Pears *(Town House)*		3
Pears, Lite *(Country Pure)*	★	
Pears, Lite *(Del Monte)*		3
Pears, Sliced *(Del Monte)*	★	
Pie Filling, Apple *(Musselman's)*		3

1 = High Fat	2 = High Sodium	3 = High Refined Sugar	5 = Cholesterol
1+ = Very High Fat	2+ = Very High Sodium	4 = Highly Processed	★= Better Choice

VARIETY *(Brand)*   RATING CODE

Variety (Brand)	Rating Code
Pie Filling, Blueberry *(Musselman's)*	3
Pie Filling, Pineapple *(Musselman's)*	3
Pineapple, Chunky, Crushed, Sliced, Tidbits & Spears *(Del Monte)*	★
Pineapple, Chunked, Crushed & Sliced *(Dole)*	★
Pineapple, Chunked, Crushed & Sliced *(3-Diamonds)*	★
Pineapple, Chunked, Crushed & Sliced *(Town House)*	★
Pineapple, Crushed & Chunks *(Rainbow)*	★
Pineapple, Sliced, Chunked & Crushed *(Liberty Gold)*	★
Plums, Mirabelles *(ReNa)*	3
Plums, Purple *(S & W)*	3
Plums, Purple *(Thank You)*	3
Plums, Purple, Whole *(Oregon)*	3
Prunes *(SunSweet)*	3
Prunes, Prepared *(S & W)*	3
Pumpkin *(Libby's)*	★
Raspberries, Red *(Oregon)*	3
Strawberries *(Fruitful)*	3
DRIED	
Apples *(Sonoma)*	★
Apricots *(Sonoma)*	★
Cherries *(Sonoma)*	★
Currants *(Sun-Maid)*	★
Dates *(Sonoma)*	★
Dates, Chopped *(Dole)*	★
Dates, Chopped *(Dromedary)*	3
Dates, Pitted *(Dole)*	★
Dates, Pitted *(Dromedary)*	★
Prunes *(Sonoma)*	★
Prunes, Pitted *(SunSweet)*	★
Raisins *(Del Monte)*	★
Raisins *(Dole)*	★
Raisins *(Dromedary)*	★
Raisins *(Sun-Maid)*	★

1 = High Fat   2 = High Sodium   3 = High Refined Sugar   5 = Cholesterol
1+ = Very High Fat   2+ = Very High Sodium   4 = Highly Processed   ★= Better Choice

VARIETY *(Brand)*   RATING CODE

VARIETY (Brand)			
FROZEN			
Blackberries *(Bel-air)*	★		
Blackberries *(Big Valley)*	★		
Blackberries *(Overlake)*	★		
Blackberries *(Stilwell)*	★		
Blackberries *(VIP)*	★		
Blackberries *(Wilderness)*	★		
Blueberries *(Big Valley)*	★		
Blueberries *(Overlake)*	★		
Blueberries *(Stilwell)*	★		
Blueberries *(Wilderness)*	★		
Cherries, Dark Sweet *(Big Valley)*	★		
Melon Balls, Mixed *(Big Valley)*	★		
Mixed Fruit *(Big Valley)*	★		
Mixed Fruit *(Stilwell)*	★		
Mixed Fruit *(Wilderness)*	★		
Peaches *(Big Valley)*	★		
Peaches *(Stilwell)*	★		
Peaches *(Wilderness)*	★		
Raspberries *(Big Valley)*	★		
Raspberries *(Overlake)*	★		
Raspberries *(VIP)*	★		
Raspberries, Sweetened *(Bel-air)*		3	
Rhubarb *(Big Valley)*	★		
Rhubarb *(Stilwell)*	★		
Strawberries *(Bel-air)*	★		
Strawberries *(Big Valley)*	★		
Strawberries *(Birds Eye)*		3	
Strawberries *(Overlake)*	★		
Strawberries *(Stilwell)*	★		
Strawberries *(VIP)*	★		
Strawberries *(Wilderness)*	★		
Strawberries & Peaches *(Bel-air)*	★		
Strawberries, Sliced *(Naturipe)*		3	

1 = High Fat	2 = High Sodium	3 = High Refined Sugar	5 = Cholesterol
1+ = Very High Fat	2+ = Very High Sodium	4 = Highly Processed	★= Better Choice

VARIETY *(Brand)*   RATING CODE

Strawberries, Sliced & Sweetened *(Bel-air)*	3
Strawberries, Sweetened *(VIP)*	3

1 = High Fat   2 = High Sodium   3 = High Refined Sugar   5 = Cholesterol
1+ = Very High Fat   2+ = Very High Sodium   4 = Highly Processed   ★= Better Choice

ICE CREAM AND OTHER FROZEN CONFECTIONS

America's favorite — and does it ever sell! I guess I'm like Will Rogers: "I never met an ice cream I didn't like." I really love the stuff, but it is not a substitute for food. Varieties with additives and preservatives (such as polysorbates, artificial color, artificial flavor, coconut oil, palm oil and NutraSweet in the diet varieties) have been eliminated.

All traditional ice creams are high in fat and sugar and some even have eggs added (extra cholesterol). The lowfat varieties and frozen yogurts are lower in fat; however, remember that as the fat content goes down, the sugar content goes up. Manufacturers have to make it taste rich some way or we wouldn't buy it. Enjoy, but do be aware of what you're getting, and limit amounts.

VARIETY *(Brand)*   RATING CODE

ICE CREAM AND OTHER FROZEN CONFECTIONS
FROZEN BARS

Variety (Brand)			
Chocolate Fudge Swirl *(Sealtest)*		3	
Fruit & Cream, Peach *(Dole)*		3	
Fruit & Cream, Strawberry *(Dole)*		3	
Fruit & Juice, Cherry *(Dole)*		3	
Fruit & Juice, Pineapple *(Dole)*		3	
Fruit & Juice, Raspberry *(Dole)*		3	
Fruit & Juice, Strawberry *(Dole)*		3	
Fudge Bar *(Häagen-Dazs)*	1	3	5
Lemon Bar *(Jell-O)*		3	
Orange *(Jell-O)*		3	
Orange & Cream *(Häagen-Dazs)*	1	3	5

FROZEN YOGURT

Variety (Brand)			
Almond Amaretto *(Brice's)*		3	
Banana Strawberry *(Dreyer's)*		3	
Banana Strawberry *(Edy's)*		3	
Black Cherry *(Sealtest)*		3	
Blueberry *(Edy's)*		3	
Blueberry *(Lucerne)*		3	
Cappuccino *(Brice's)*		3	
Cherry *(Dreyer's)*		3	
Cherry *(Edy's)*		3	
Cherry *(Lucerne)*		3	
Chocolate *(Breyers)*		3	
Chocolate *(Brice's)*		3	
Chocolate *(Dreyer's)*		3	
Chocolate *(Edy's)*		3	
Chocolate Amaretto *(Koala Kreme)*		3	5
French Vanilla *(Koala Kreme)*		3	5
Hokey Pokey *(Koala Kreme)*	1	3	5
Macadamia Nut *(Koala Kreme)*	1	3	5
Milk Chocolate *(Homemade)*		3	
Peach *(Blue Bunny)*		3	
Peach *(Edy's)*		3	

1 = High Fat   2 = High Sodium   3 = High Refined Sugar   5 = Cholesterol
1+ = Very High Fat   2+ = Very High Sodium   4 = Highly Processed   ★= Better Choice

VARIETY *(Brand)*   RATING CODE

Peach *(Homemade)*		3	
Peach *(Lucerne)*		3	
Peach *(Rhapsody Farms)*		3	
Peach *(Sealtest)*		3	
Raspberry *(Lucerne)*		3	
Red Raspberry *(Breyers)*		3	
Strawberry *(Breyers)*		3	
Strawberry *(Brice's)*		3	
Strawberry *(Dreyer's)*		3	
Strawberry *(Edy's)*		3	
Strawberry *(Homemade)*		3	
Strawberry *(Lucerne)*		3	
Strawberry *(Sealtest)*		3	
Vanilla *(Breyers)*		3	
Vanilla *(Edy's)*		3	
Vanilla *(Homemade)*		3	
Vanilla *(Lucerne)*		3	
Vanilla *(Rhapsody Farms)*		3	
ICE CREAM			
Almond Praline *(Edy's)*	1+	3	5
Black Cherry, Fat Free *(Borden)*		3	
Butter Pecan *(Breyers)*	1+	3	5
Butter Pecan *(Edy's)*	1+	3	5
Butter Pecan *(Homemade)*	1	3	5
Butter Pecan *(Swensen's)*	1+	3	5
Cafe Amaretto *(Steve's)*	1+	3	5
Cappuccino *(Rice Dream)*	1		
Caramel Apple *(Edy's)*	1+	3	5
Carob Almond *(Rice Dream)*	1		
Cherry *(Breyers)*	1	3	5
Cherry Vanilla *(Breyers)*	1	3	5
Chocolate *(Ben & Jerry's)*	1+	3	5
Chocolate *(Breyers)*	1	3	5
Chocolate *(Dreyer's)*	1+	3	5

1 = High Fat	2 = High Sodium	3 = High Refined Sugar 5 = Cholesterol
1+ = Very High Fat	2+ = Very High Sodium	4 = Highly Processed ★= Better Choice

VARIETY (Brand)   RATING CODE

VARIETY (Brand)			
Chocolate *(Homemade)*	1	3	5
Chocolate *(Pet)*	1	3	5
Chocolate Chip *(Edy's)*	1+	3	5
Chocolate Chip *(Swensen's)*	1+	3	5
Chocolate Chocolate Chip *(Edy's)*	1+	3	5
Chocolate Fudge Mousse *(Edy's)*	1+	3	5
Chocolate, Fat Free *(Borden)*		3	
Chocolate, Heavy Belgian *(Steve's)*	1+	3	5
Cocoa Marble Fudge *(Rice Dream)*	★		
Creamy Caramel Nut *(Dreyer's)*	1+	3	5
Dastardly Mash *(Ben & Jerry's)*	1+	3	5
Dutch Chocolate *(Blue Bell)*	1	3	5
Dutch Chocolate with Almond *(Homemade)*	1	3	5
Extra Light Peach *(Blue Bell)*		3	
Extra Light Strawberry *(Blue Bell)*		3	
French Vanilla *(Ben & Jerry's)*	1+	3	5
French Vanilla *(Dreyer's)*	1+	3	5
French Vanilla *(Edy's)*	1+	3	5
French Vanilla *(Steve's)*	1+	3	5
Hawaiian Sundae *(Homemade)*	1	3	5
Lemon *(Rice Dream)*	1		
Light, Almond Praline *(Edy's)*	1	3	
Light, Banana Politan *(Edy's)*	1	3	
Light, Butter Pecan *(Edy's)*	1	3	
Light, Butter Pecan *(Steve's)*	1	3	5
Light, Cafe au Lait *(Dreyer's)*	1	3	5
Light, Cafe au Lait *(Edy's)*	1	3	
Light, Cherry Chocolate Chunk *(Steve's)*	1	3	5
Light, Chocolate *(Breyers)*		3	
Light, Chocolate Fudge Mousse *(Dreyer's)*	1	3	
Light, Marble Fudge *(Dreyer's)*		3	
Light, Marble Fudge *(Edy's)*		3	
Light, Peanut Butter & Chocolate *(Edy's)*	1	3	

1 = High Fat   2 = High Sodium   3 = High Refined Sugar   5 = Cholesterol
1+ = Very High Fat   2+ = Very High Sodium   4 = Highly Processed   ★= Better Choice

VARIETY *(Brand)* — RATING CODE

VARIETY (Brand)	1	3	5
Light, Raspberry *(Dreyer's)*	1	3	5
Light, Rocky Road *(Dreyer's)*	1	3	
Light, Rocky Road *(Edy's)*	1	3	
Light, Strawberry *(Breyers)*		3	
Light, Strawberry *(Dreyer's)*	1	3	5
Light, Strawberry *(Edy's)*	1	3	
Light, Vanilla *(Breyers)*		3	
Light, Vanilla *(Dreyer's)*	1	3	
Light, Vanilla *(Edy's)*	1	3	
Light, Vanilla *(Steve's)*	1	3	5
Marble Fudge *(Edy's)*	1+	3	5
Mocha Almond Fudge *(Dreyer's)*	1+	3	5
Mocha Almond Fudge *(Edy's)*	1+	3	5
Natural Vanilla Bean *(Blue Bell)*	1	3	5
New York Super Fudge Chunk *(Ben & Jerry's)*	1+	3	5
Peach *(Breyers)*	1	3	5
Peach, Fat Free *(Borden)*		3	
Peaches 'n Cream *(Homemade)*	1	3	5
Peanut Butter Fudge *(Rice Dream)*	1		
Rocky Road *(Dreyer's)*	1+	3	5
Rocky Road *(Edy's)*	1+	3	5
Rocky Road *(Swensen's)*	1+	3	5
Strawberries 'n Cream *(Homemade)*	1	3	5
Strawberry *(Blue Bell)*	1	3	5
Strawberry *(Breyers)*	1	3	5
Strawberry *(Rice Dream)*	1		
Strawberry, Fat Free *(Borden)*		3	
Vanilla *(Breyers)*	1	3	5
Vanilla *(Dreyer's)*	1+	3	5
Vanilla *(Edy's)*	1+	3	5
Vanilla *(Homemade)*	1	3	5
Vanilla *(Swensen's)*	1+	3	5
Vanilla Fudge Twirl *(Breyers)*	1	3	5

1 = High Fat   2 = High Sodium   3 = High Refined Sugar   5 = Cholesterol
1+ = Very High Fat   2+ = Very High Sodium   4 = Highly Processed   ★= Better Choice

VARIETY (Brand)

RATING CODE

Vanilla, Single Cups (Homemade)	1	3	5
Vanilla Chocolate Strawberry (Dreyer's)	1+	3	5
Vanilla Chocolate Strawberry (Edy's)	1+	3	5
Wild Berry (Rice Dream)	1		
SORBET			
Blueberry Cream (Häagen-Dazs)	1	3	5
Key Lime (Häagen-Dazs)	1	3	5
Mandarin (Dole)		3	
Orange & Cream (Häagen-Dazs)	1	3	5
Peach (Dole)		3	
Pineapple (Dole)		3	
Raspberry (Steve's)		3	
Raspberry & Cream (Häagen-Dazs)	1	3	5
Strawberry (Dole)		3	
OTHER			
Ice Bean, Carob Chip (Farm Foods)	1+	3	
Ice Bean, Cherry Vanilla (Farm Foods)	1+	3	
Ice Bean, Heavenly Hash (Farm Foods)	1+	3	
Ice Bean, Honey Vanilla (Farm Foods)	1+	3	
Ice Bean, Toasted Almond Fudge (Farm Foods)	1+	3	
Nice Dream, Butter Fudge (Rice Dream)	1		
Rice Dream, Cappuccino (Rice Dream)	1		
Rice Dream, Carob Almond (Rice Dream)	1		
Rice Dream, Cocoa Marble Fudge (Rice Dream)	★		
Rice Dream, Lemon (Rice Dream)	1		
Rice Dream, Strawberry (Rice Dream)	1		
Rice Dream, Wildberry (Rice Dream)	1		
Tofruzen, Chocolate Chip (Tofruzen)	1	3	
Tofruzen, Maple Toffee Chip (Tofruzen)	1	3	
Tofruzen, Mountain Berry (Tofruzen)	1	3	
Tofruzen, Peach Amaretto (Tofruzen)	1	3	
Tofruzen, Praline Pecan (Tofruzen)	1	3	
Tofruzen, Strawberry (Tofruzen)	1	3	

1 = High Fat	2 = High Sodium	3 = High Refined Sugar	5 = Cholesterol
1+ = Very High Fat	2+ = Very High Sodium	4 = Highly Processed	★= Better Choice

VARIETY (Brand)   RATING CODE

Tofruzen, Vanilla Almond (Tofruzen)	1	3
Tofutti, Almond Bark (Tofutti)	1+	3
Tofutti, Butter Pecan (Tofutti)	1+	3
Tofutti, Chocolate (Tofutti)		3
Tofutti, Chocolate Supreme (Tofutti)	1+	3
Tofutti, Chocolate Cookies Supreme (Tofutti)	1+	3
Tofutti, Deep Chocolate Fudge (Tofutti)	1+	3
Tofutti, Lite lite Chocolate Vanilla Twirl (Tofutti)		3
Tofutti, Wildberry Supreme (Tofutti)	1+	3

1 = High Fat   2 = High Sodium   3 = High Refined Sugar   5 = Cholesterol
1+ = Very High Fat   2+ = Very High Sodium   4 = Highly Processed   ★= Better Choice

JELLIES, JAMS, PRESERVES AND HONEY

There are numerous products in this category. Most all are free of additives and preservatives, with the exception of some low-calorie jams and jellies. For example: *Smucker's* Low-Sugar Strawberry Spread contains potassium sorbate and artificial color. Most all "regular" varieties are high in refined sugar; however, we are seeing more and more products which contain only fruit and fruit juice as their source of sweeteners. These are the best choices. They are high in sugar content, but it is not refined sugar.

As for honey, it is a highly refined sugar (the bees do the refining); however, since honey is sweeter than white table sugar, it takes less to achieve the same results.

Want a dessert that is nutritious and tasty? Get some plain nonfat yogurt, add some *Smucker's* Simply Fruit Preserves and a sliced ripe banana. This one will grow on you!

VARIETY *(Brand)*   RATING CODE

JELLIES, JAMS, PRESERVES AND HONEY
JELLIES, JAMS AND PRESERVES

Variety (Brand)	Rating Code
Apple *(Griffin's)*	3
Apple *(Kraft)*	3
Apple Butter *(Eden)*	★
Apple Butter *(Garden Club)*	3
Apple Butter *(Griffin's)*	3
Apple Butter *(L & A)*	★
Apple Butter *(Musselman's)*	3
Apple Butter *(New Morning)*	★
Apple Butter *(R. W. Knudsen)*	★
Apple Butter *(Shiloh Farms)*	★
Apple Butter, Simply Fruit *(Smucker's)*	★
Apple Butter, Spiced Cider *(Smucker's)*	3
Apple Grape, Squeezable *(Welch's)*	3
Apple Spread *(Poiret)*	★
Apricot *(Bama)*	3
Apricot *(Chambord)*	3
Apricot *(European Royalty)*	3
Apricot *(Garden Club)*	3
Apricot *(Griffin's)*	3
Apricot *(Knott's Berry Farm)*	3
Apricot *(Kraft)*	3
Apricot *(Nelson's)*	3
Apricot *(Polaner)*	★
Apricot *(Smucker's)*	3
Apricot *(Sorrell Ridge)*	★
Apricot Pineapple *(Knott's Berry Farm)*	3
Apricot Pineapple *(R. W. Knudsen)*	★
Apricot Spread *(Poiret)*	★
Apricot, Simply Fruit *(Smucker's)*	★
Berry, Wild *(Knott's Berry Farm)*	3
Black Cherry *(Poiret)*	★
Black Cherry *(Polaner)*	★
Black Cherry *(R. W. Knudsen)*	★

1 = High Fat   2 = High Sodium   3 = High Refined Sugar   5 = Cholesterol
1+ = Very High Fat   2+ = Very High Sodium   4 = Highly Processed   ★= Better Choice

VARIETY *(Brand)*   RATING CODE

Black Cherry *(Sorrell Ridge)*	★	
Black Raspberry *(Sorrell Ridge)*	★	
Blackberry *(Bonne Maman)*		3
Blackberry *(Garden Club)*		3
Blackberry *(Griffin's)*		3
Blackberry *(Knott's Berry Farm)*		3
Blackberry *(Kraft)*		3
Blackberry *(Polaner)*	★	
Blackberry *(R. W. Knudsen)*	★	
Blackberry *(Smucker's)*		3
Blackberry *(Sorrell Ridge)*	★	
Blackberry, Simply Fruit *(Smucker's)*	★	
Blueberry *(Knott's Berry Farm)*		3
Blueberry *(Polaner)*	★	
Blueberry *(R. W. Knudsen)*	★	
Blueberry *(Sorrell Ridge)*	★	
Blueberry Conserve *(Cascadian Farm)*		3
Blueberry, Simply Fruit *(Smucker's)*	★	
Boysenberry *(Knott's Berry Farm)*		3
Boysenberry *(R. W. Knudsen)*	★	
Boysenberry *(Sorrell Ridge)*	★	
Cherry *(European Royalty)*		3
Cherry *(Smucker's)*		3
Cherry *(Sorrell Ridge)*	★	
Cherry Orange *(Sorrell Ridge)*	★	
Cherry, Bing *(Knott's Berry Farm)*		3
Cherry, Red *(Knott's Berry Farm)*		3
Concord Grape *(R. W. Knudsen)*	★	
Concord Grape *(Sorrell Ridge)*	★	
Crabapple *(Knott's Berry Farm)*		3
Cranberry *(Sorrell Ridge)*	★	
Cranberry Orange *(Patti's)*		3
Cranberry Strawberry *(Patti's)*		3

1 = High Fat	2 = High Sodium	3 = High Refined Sugar	5 = Cholesterol
1+ = Very High Fat	2+ = Very High Sodium	4 = Highly Processed	★= Better Choice

VARIETY *(Brand)*   RATING CODE

VARIETY (Brand)	RATING CODE
Currant *(Smucker's)*	3
Currant, Red *(Knott's Berry Farm)*	3
Fig *(Braswell's)*	3
Fig, Kadota *(Knott's Berry Farm)*	3
Grape *(Bama)*	3
Grape *(Garden Club)*	3
Grape *(Griffin's)*	3
Grape *(Knott's Berry Farm)*	3
Grape *(Kraft)*	3
Grape *(Polaner)*	★
Grape *(Rainbow)*	3
Grape *(Smucker's)*	3
Grape *(Welch's)*	3
Grape, Simply Fruit *(Smucker's)*	★
Grape, Squeeze *(Welch's)*	3
Guava *(Crosse & Blackwell)*	3
Jalapeño *(Gourmet Award)*	3
Marmalade *(Bama)*	3
Marmalade *(Bonne Maman)*	3
Marmalade *(Knott's Berry Farm)*	3
Marmalade *(Smucker's)*	3
Marmalade, Simply Fruit *(Smucker's)*	★
Mixed Fruit *(European Royalty)*	3
Orange *(Polaner)*	★
Orange Marmalade *(R. W. Knudsen)*	★
Orange Marmalade *(Sorrell Ridge)*	★
Peach *(Bama)*	3
Peach *(Bonne Maman)*	3
Peace *(European Royalty)*	3
Peach *(Garden Club)*	3
Peach *(Griffin's)*	3
Peach *(Knott's Berry Farm)*	3
Peach *(Kraft)*	3

1 = High Fat	2 = High Sodium	3 = High Refined Sugar	5 = Cholesterol
1+ = Very High Fat	2+ = Very High Sodium	4 = Highly Processed	★= Better Choice

VARIETY *(Brand)*   RATING CODE

Variety (Brand)	Rating Code
Peach *(Polaner)*	★
Peach *(R. W. Knudsen)*	★
Peach *(Smucker's)*	3
Peach *(Sorrell Ridge)*	★
Peach Butter *(Braswell's)*	3
Peach Butter *(Smucker's)*	3
Pear *(Braswell's)*	3
Pear & Lemon *(Poiret)*	★
Pear & Orange *(Poiret)*	★
Pear & Passion Fruit *(Poiret)*	★
Pineapple *(Garden Club)*	3
Pineapple *(Griffin's)*	3
Pineapple *(Sorrell Ridge)*	★
Plum *(European Royalty)*	3
Plum Good *(Sorrell Ridge)*	★
Plum, California *(Knott's Berry Farm)*	3
Plum, Red *(Bama)*	3
Plum, Red *(Griffin's)*	3
Plum, Red *(Smucker's)*	3
Raspberry *(Bonne Maman)*	3
Raspberry *(European Royalty)*	3
Raspberry *(Poiret)*	★
Raspberry *(Sorrell Ridge)*	★
Raspberry Conserve *(Cascadian Farm)*	3
Raspberry, Black *(Smucker's)*	3
Raspberry, Red *(Knott's Berry Farm)*	3
Raspberry, Red *(Polaner)*	★
Raspberry, Red *(Smucker's)*	3
Raspberry, Simply Fruit *(Smucker's)*	★
Red Currant Raspberry *(Bonne Maman)*	3
Red Raspberry *(R. W. Knudsen)*	★
Rhubarb Raspberry *(Braswell's)*	3
Seedless Raspberry *(Sorrell Ridge)*	★

1 = High Fat	2 = High Sodium	3 = High Refined Sugar	5 = Cholesterol
1+ = Very High Fat	2+ = Very High Sodium	4 = Highly Processed	★= Better Choice

VARIETY *(Brand)*   RATING CODE

Variety (Brand)	★	Rating
Strawberry *(Bama)*		3
Strawberry *(European Royalty)*		3
Strawberry *(Fruitful)*		3
Strawberry *(Garden Club)*		3
Strawberry *(Griffin's)*		3
Strawberry *(Knott's Berry Farm)*		3
Strawberry *(Kraft)*		3
Strawberry *(Poiret)*	★	
Strawberry *(Polaner)*	★	
Strawberry *(R. W. Knudsen)*	★	
Strawberry *(Rainbow)*		3
Strawberry *(Smucker's)*		3
Strawberry *(Sorrell Ridge)*	★	
Strawberry Conserve *(Cascadian Farm)*		3
Strawberry Rhubarb *(Sorrell Ridge)*	★	
Strawberry, Fresh Pack *(Smucker's)*		3
Strawberry, Natural *(Smucker's)*		3
Strawberry, Simply Fruit *(Smucker's)*	★	
Strawberry, Squeeze *(Welch's)*		3
3 Pepper, Spicy *(Patti's)*		3
Tomato *(Knott's Berry Farm)*		3

HONEY

Variety (Brand)	Rating
Honey *(Arthur Nokes)*	3 4
Honey *(Burleson's)*	3 4
Honey *(Clover Maid)*	3 4
Honey *(Joe's Honey)*	3 4
Honey *(Ozarka)*	3 4
Honey *(Rainbow)*	3 4
Honey *(Walker's)*	3 4
Honey, Clover *(Dutch Gold)*	3 4
Honey, Clover *(Sue Bee)*	3 4
Honey, Creamed *(Burleson's)*	3 4
Honey, Raw *(Aunt Sue's)*	3 4
Honey, Raw *(Cheatwood's)*	3 4

1 = High Fat 2 = High Sodium 3 = High Refined Sugar 5 = Cholesterol
1+ = Very High Fat 2+ = Very High Sodium 4 = Highly Processed ★= Better Choice

VARIETY *(Brand)*	RATING CODE
Honey, Spun *(Sue Bee)*	3 4
Honey, Wild & Unfiltered *(Tropical)*	3 4

JUICES

To make it easier for you, I have divided juice into different categories; bottled, canned, frozen and refrigerated. I have some very strong feelings about juices. Of course, juice without refined sugar is the best choice; but more importantly, when a fruit or vegetable is processed into a juice, it looses a high percentage of its vitamins and minerals as well as its fiber. In other words, a fresh or frozen fruit or vegetable is always a better choice than the juice.

I know that convenience plays a big part here; so when choosing juices those with the pulp are the best choices. As for additives and preservatives, 100% real juice rarely contains them. White grape juice is an exception as some contain sulfites. Two products that I see people using are *non-refrigerated Real Lemon juice* and *boxed juices*. The Real Lemon contains sodium benzoate and sodium bisulfite, and the boxed juices are lined with aluminum. I don't like any juice in contact with aluminum. As for the juice drinks, punches, etc., I don't rate them much over soda pop, and many contain additives and preservatives.

VARIETY *(Brand)*   RATING CODE

JUICES
BOTTLED
Almond Nectar *(Lakewood)*   ★
Ambrosia *(R. W. Knudsen)*   ★
Apple *(After the Fall)*   ★

Apple *(Apple & Eve)*   ★
Apple *(Carolina Classic)*   ★
Apple *(Carolina Gold)*   ★

Apple *(Hansen's)*   ★
Apple *(Indian Summer)*   ★
Apple *(Martinelli's)*   ★

Apple *(Mott's)*   ★
Apple *(Musselman's)*   ★
Apple *(R. W. Knudsen)*   ★

Apple *(Rainbow)*   ★
Apple *(S & W)*   ★
Apple *(Santa Cruz Natural)*   ★

Apple *(Seneca)*   ★
Apple *(Skyland)*   ★
Apple *(Speas Farm)*   ★

Apple *(Thank You)*   ★
Apple *(Town House)*   ★
Apple *(Tree of Life)*   ★

Apple *(Tree Top)*   ★
Apple *(White House)*   ★
Apple *(Wilderness)*   ★

Apple Cider *(Indian Summer)*   ★
Apple Cider *(Martinelli's)*   ★
Apple Cider *(Mott's)*   ★

Apple Cider *(Musselman's)*   ★
Apple Cider *(Tree Top)*   ★
Apple Cider *(Town House)*   ★

Apple Cider *(Wilderness)*   ★
Apple Clear *(R. W. Knudsen)*   ★
Apple Juice, Old-Fashioned *(Heinke's)*   ★

VARIETY *(Brand)*   RATING CODE

VARIETY (Brand)	RATING CODE
Apple Juice, Unfiltered *(Martinelli's)*	★
Apple Juice, Unfiltered *(Tree Top)*	★
Apple, Gravenstein *(R. W. Knudsen)*	★
Apple, Mountain *(Mountain Sun)*	★
Apple, Natural *(R. W. Knudsen)*	★
Apple, Organic *(Mountain Sun)*	★
Apple-Apricot *(Looza)*	3
Apple-Apricot *(R. W. Knudsen)*	★
Apple-Banana *(R. W. Knudsen)*	★
Apple-Blackberry *(R. W. Knudsen)*	★
Apple-Blackberry *(Santa Cruz Natural)*	★
Apple-Boysenberry *(R. W. Knudsen)*	★
Apple-Boysenberry *(Santa Cruz Natural)*	★
Apple-Cherry *(Looza)*	3
Apple-Cranberry *(Apple & Eve)*	★
Apple-Cranberry *(R. W. Knudsen)*	★
Apple-Cranberry *(Town House)*	3
Apple-Grape *(Tree Top)*	★
Apple-Grape *(Welch's Orchard)*	3
Apple-Orange-Pineapple *(Welch's Orchard)*	3
Apple-Peach *(R. W. Knudsen)*	★
Apple-Pear *(Tree Top)*	★
Apple-Raspberry *(R. W. Knudsen)*	★
Apple-Raspberry *(Mountain Sun)*	★
Apple-Strawberry *(R. W. Knudsen)*	★
Apple-Strawberry *(Santa Cruz Natural)*	★
Apple-Strawberry *(Tree of Life)*	★
Apricot Nectar *(Looza)*	3
Apricot Nectar *(R. W. Knudsen)*	★
Apricot Nectar *(Santa Cruz Natural)*	★
Banana Nectar *(Looza)*	3
Black Cherry *(R. W. Knudsen)*	★
Blueberry Nectar *(R. W. Knudsen)*	★

1 = High Fat   2 = High Sodium   3 = High Refined Sugar   5 = Cholesterol
1+ = Very High Fat   2+ = Very High Sodium   4 = Highly Processed   ★= Better Choice

VARIETY *(Brand)*   RATING CODE

Variety (Brand)	Rating
Blueberry Premier *(R. W. Knudsen)*	★
Boysenberry *(R. W. Knudsen)*	★
Boysenberry Nectar *(R. W. Knudsen)*	★
Boysenberry Punch *(After the Fall)*	★
Breakfast Juice, Natural *(R. W. Knudsen)*	★
California Twist *(Heinke's)*	★
Carrot *(Hollywood)*	★
Cherry *(Mountain Sun)*	★
Cherry Cider *(Heinke's)*	★
Cherry Cider *(Mountain Sun)*	★
Cherry Cider *(R. W. Knudsen)*	★
Cherry Lemonade *(Santa Cruz Natural)*	3
Cherry Premier *(R. W. Knudsen)*	★
Cider & Spice *(R. W. Knudsen)*	★
Cider & Spice *(Mountain Sun)*	★
Concord Grape *(Heinke's)*	★
Concord Grape *(Mountain Sun)*	★
Concord Grape *(R. W. Knudsen)*	★
Concord Grape *(Tree of Life)*	★
Country Raspberry, Pure & Light *(Dole)*	★
Cran-Apple *(Ocean Spray)*	3
Cran-Apple Delight *(L & A)*	★
Cran-Blueberry *(Ocean Spray)*	3
Cran-Grape *(Ocean Spray)*	3
Cran-Raspberry *(Ocean Spray)*	3
Cran-Strawberry *(Ocean Spray)*	3
Cranberry *(Mountain Home)*	★
Cranberry *(R. W. Knudsen)*	★
Cranberry *(Smucker's)*	★
Cranberry Apple *(Rainbow)*	3
Cranberry Blueberry *(R. W. Knudsen)*	★
Cranberry Grape *(Apple & Eve)*	★
Cranberry Juice Cocktail *(Maxxi)*	3

1 = High Fat	2 = High Sodium	3 = High Refined Sugar	5 = Cholesterol
1+ = Very High Fat	2+ = Very High Sodium	4 = Highly Processed	★= Better Choice

VARIETY *(Brand)*   RATING CODE

	★	3		
Cranberry Juice Cocktail *(Ocean Spray)*		3		
Cranberry Juice Cocktail *(Town House)*		3		
Cranberry Meets Raspberry *(After the Fall)*	★			
Cranberry Nectar *(Heinke's)*	★			
Cranberry Nectar *(R. W. Knudsen)*	★			
Cranberry Premier *(R. W. Knudsen)*	★			
Cranberry Raspberry *(R. W. Knudsen)*	★			
Cranberry, Cape Cod *(After the Fall)*	★			
Cranberry, Naturally *(Apple & Eve)*	★			
Cranicot *(Ocean Spray)*		3		
Cream Papaya *(R. W. Knudsen)*	★			
Grape *(R. W. Knudsen)*	★			
Grape *(Seneca)*	★			
Grape *(Town House)*	★			
Grape *(Welch's Orchard)*		3		
Grape Blackberry Lemonade *(Santa Cruz Natural)*		3		
Grape Juice, Cocktail *(Welch's Orchard)*		3		
Grape, Purple Only *(Welch's)*	★			
Grapefruit *(R. W. Knudsen)*	★			
Grapefruit *(Ocean Spray)*	★			
Grapefruit *(Tree Sweet)*	★			
Grapefruit Orange *(Texsun)*		3		
Guava Strawberry *(Smucker's)*	★			
Guava, Tropicals *(Welch's Orchard)*		3		
Harvest Blend *(Welch's Orchard)*		3		
Hibiscus *(Mountain Sun)*	★			
Hibiscus Cooler *(R. W. Knudsen)*	★			
Kiwi Nectar *(R. W. Knudsen)*	★			
Koala Punch *(After the Fall)*	★			
Lemon *(Mountain Sun)*	★			
Lemon *(R. W. Knudsen)*	★			
Lemonade *(After the Fall)*	★			
Lemonade *(Santa Cruz Natural)*		3		

1 = High Fat	2 = High Sodium	3 = High Refined Sugar	5 = Cholesterol
1+ = Very High Fat	2+ = Very High Sodium	4 = Highly Processed	★= Better Choice

VARIETY *(Brand)*   RATING CODE

Variety (Brand)	★		3	
Lemonade, Cherry *(R. W. Knudsen)*	★			
Lemonade, Cranberry *(R. W. Knudsen)*	★			
Lemonade, Natural *(R. W. Knudsen)*	★			
Lemonade, Raspberry *(After the Fall)*	★			
Lemonade, Raspberry *(R. W. Knudsen)*	★			
Lemonade, Strawberry *(R. W. Knudsen)*	★			
Mandarin Tangerine, Pure & Light *(Dole)*	★			
Martha's Vineyard Garden Blend *(After the Fall)*	★			
Martha's Vineyard Grape *(After the Fall)*	★			
Mauna La'i Guava Fruit Drink *(Ocean Spray)*			3	
Mauna La'i Guava Passion Fruit Drink *(Ocean Spray)*			3	
Mountain Cherry, Pure & Light *(Dole)*	★			
Orange *(R. W. Knudsen)*	★			
Orange-Apricot *(Tropicana Twister)*			3	
Orange-Mango *(R. W. Knudsen)*	★			
Orange-Passion Fruit *(Tropicana Twister)*			3	
Orange-Strawberry-Banana *(Tropicana Twister)*			3	
Orchard Peach, Pure & Light *(Dole)*	★			
Oregon Berry *(After the Fall)*	★			
Papaya *(Mountain Sun)*	★			
Papaya Nectar *(R. W. Knudsen)*	★			
Papaya Nectar Concentrate *(R. W. Knudsen)*	★			
Papaya-Pineapple *(L & A)*	★			
Parrot's Punch *(After the Fall)*	★			
Passion *(Mountain Sun)*	★			
Passion Fruit Nectar *(Looza)*			3	
Passion Fruit Raspberry *(Smucker's)*	★			
Passion Fruit Tropicals *(Welch's Orchard)*			3	
Peach *(Mountain Sun)*	★			
Peach *(Smucker's)*	★			
Peach Nectar *(After the Fall)*	★			
Peach Nectar *(Looza)*			3	
Peach Nectar *(R. W. Knudsen)*	★			

1 = High Fat   2 = High Sodium   3 = High Refined Sugar   5 = Cholesterol
1+ = Very High Fat   2+ = Very High Sodium   4 = Highly Processed   ★= Better Choice

VARIETY *(Brand)*   RATING CODE

Peach Premier *(R. W. Knudsen)*	★
Pear *(After the Fall)*	★
Pear *(Heinke's)*	★

Pear *(R. W. Knudsen)*	★
Pear Nectar *(After the Fall)*	★
Pear Nectar *(Looza)*	3

Pineapple *(R. W. Knudsen)*	★
Pineapple Banana, Tropicals *(Welch's Orchard)*	3
Pineapple Grapefruit *(Tropicana Twister)*	3

Pineapple Nectar *(Lakewood)*	★
Pink Grapefruit *(R. W. Knudsen)*	★
Pink Grapefruit *(Tree Sweet)*	★

Pink Grapefruit Cocktail *(Ocean Spray)*	3
Pink Grapefruit Cocktail *(Tree Sweet)*	3
Pomegranate *(R. W. Knudsen)*	★

Prune *(Del Monte)*	★
Prune *(Mott's)*	★
Prune *(SunSweet)*	★

Prune *(Tree of Life)*	★
Prune Juice, Country Style *(Mott's)*	★
Prune, Homestyle with Pulp *(SunSweet)*	★

Raspberry *(Mountain Sun)*	★
Raspberry Cranberry *(Apple & Eve)*	★
Raspberry Lemonade *(Santa Cruz Natural)*	3

Raspberry Nectar *(R. W. Knudsen)*	★
Raspberry Peach *(R. W. Knudsen)*	★
Raspberry Premier *(R. W. Knudsen)*	★

Razzleberry *(R. W. Knudsen)*	★
Red Grape *(Welch's)*	★
Red Raspberry Nectar *(R. W. Knudsen)*	★

Riesling *(R. W. Knudsen)*	★
Snap•E•Tom, Chili Cocktail *(Snap•E•Tom)*	2+
Strawberry *(Mountain Sun)*	★

1 = High Fat	2 = High Sodium	3 = High Refined Sugar	5 = Cholesterol
1+ = Very High Fat	2+ = Very High Sodium	4 = Highly Processed	★= Better Choice

VARIETY *(Brand)*   RATING CODE

Variety (Brand)	★	1/1+	2/2+	3	
Strawberry Banana *(R. W. Knudsen)*	★				
Strawberry Cooler *(After the Fall)*	★				
Strawberry Guava *(R. W. Knudsen)*	★				
Strawberry Guava Nectar *(Santa Cruz Natural)*				3	
Strawberry Lemonade *(Santa Cruz Natural)*				3	
Strawberry Nectar *(R. W. Knudsen)*	★				
Tangerine *(R. W. Knudsen)*	★				
Three Berry Nectar *(Lakewood)*	★				
Tomato *(Campbell's)*			2+		
Tomato *(Tree of Life)*			2+		
Tomato *(Welch's)*			2		
Tropical Passion *(R. W. Knudsen)*	★				
Tropical Punch *(R. W. Knudsen)*	★				
V-8 Vegetable *(V-8)*			2+		
V-8 Vegetable, No Salt *(V-8)*	★				
V-8 Vegetable, Spicy Hot *(V-8)*			2+		
Vegetable *(Apple & Eve)*			2		
Very Veggie *(R. W. Knudsen)*			2+		
Very Veggie, Low Sodium *(R. W. Knudsen)*	★				
Very Veggie, Spicy *(R. W. Knudsen)*			2+		
Vita Juice *(R. W. Knudsen)*	★				
Watermelon Twist *(Heinke's)*	★				
White Zinfandel *(R. W. Knudsen)*	★				
CANNED					
Apple *(Big Tex)*	★				
Apple *(Musselman's)*	★				
Apple *(Seneca)*	★				
Apple *(Speas Farm)*	★				
Apple *(Town House)*	★				
Apple *(Tree Top)*	★				
Apricot Nectar *(Kern's)*				3	
Apricot Nectar *(Libby's)*				3	
Apricot Nectar *(S & W)*				3	

1 = High Fat	2 = High Sodium	3 = High Refined Sugar	5 = Cholesterol
1+ = Very High Fat	2+ = Very High Sodium	4 = Highly Processed	★= Better Choice

VARIETY *(Brand)*   RATING CODE

VARIETY (Brand)	★	2+	3
Apricot Nectar *(Town House)*			3
Banana Pineapple Nectar *(Kern's)*			3
Carrot *(Hollywood)*	★		
Grape *(Welch's)*	★		
Grapefruit *(Big Tex)*	★		
Grapefruit *(Del Monte)*	★		
Grapefruit *(Donald Duck)*	★		
Grapefruit *(Ocean Spray)*	★		
Grapefruit *(Old South)*	★		
Grapefruit *(Town House)*	★		
Juicy Juice Berry *(Libby's)*	★		
Juicy Juice, Cherry *(Libby's)*	★		
Juicy Juice, Grape *(Libby's)*	★		
Juicy Juice, Punch *(Libby's)*	★		
Juicy Juice, Tropical *(Libby's)*	★		
Kraut *(Meeter's)*		2+	
Mango Nectar *(Faraon)*			3
Mango Nectar *(Kern's)*			3
Orange *(Big Tex)*	★		
Orange *(Del Monte)*	★		
Orange *(Donald Duck)*	★		
Orange *(Sunbright)*	★		
Orange *(Texsun)*	★		
Orange Pineapple *(Texsun)*			3
Papaya Nectar *(Faraon)*			3
Papaya Nectar *(Kern's)*			3
Peach Nectar *(Kern's)*			3
Peach Nectar *(Libby's)*			3
Pear Nectar *(Kern's)*			3
Pear Nectar *(Libby's)*			3
Pine-Orange-Banana *(Dole)*	★		
Pineapple *(Del Monte)*	★		
Pineapple *(Dole)*	★		

1 = High Fat   2 = High Sodium   3 = High Refined Sugar   5 = Cholesterol
1+ = Very High Fat   2+ = Very High Sodium   4 = Highly Processed   ★= Better Choice

VARIETY *(Brand)*   RATING CODE

Variety (Brand)			
Pineapple *(S & W)*	★		
Pineapple *(Town House)*	★		
Pink Grapefruit *(Donald Duck)*		3	
Pink Grapefruit *(Juice Bowl)*	★		
Pink Grapefruit *(Sunbright)*	★		
Pink Grapefruit *(Texsun)*	★		
Pink Grapefruit *(Town House)*	★		
Pink Grapefruit Cocktail *(Texsun)*		3	
Prune *(SunSweet)*	★		
Sauerkraut *(S & W)*	2+		
Snap•E•Tom, Chili Cocktail *(Snap•E•Tom)*	2+		
Tomato *(Campbell's)*	2+		
Tomato *(Del Monte)*	2+		
Tomato *(Hunt's)*	2+		
Tomato *(Libby's)*	2+		
Tomato *(Rainbow)*	2+		
Tomato *(Sacramento)*	2+		
Tomato *(Town House)*	2+		
Tomato, No Salt *(Hunt's)*	★		
V-8 Vegetable *(V-8)*	2+		
V-8 Vegetable, No Salt *(V-8)*	★		
V-8 Vegetable, Spicy Hot *(V-8)*	2+		
FROZEN			
Apple *(Bel-air)*	★		
Apple *(Minute Maid)*	★		
Apple *(Musselman's)*	★		
Apple *(Seneca)*	★		
Apple *(Tree Top)*	★		
Apple Cider *(Hardin)*	★		
Apple Cranberry *(Tree Top)*	★		
Apple Punch *(Minute Maid)*		3	
Apple, Granny Smith *(Seneca)*	★		

1 = High Fat	2 = High Sodium	3 = High Refined Sugar	5 = Cholesterol
1+ = Very High Fat	2+ = Very High Sodium	4 = Highly Processed	★= Better Choice

VARIETY *(Brand)* — RATING CODE

Variety (Brand)	Rating Code
Apple, Natural *(Seneca)*	★
Apple-Grape *(Welch's Orchard)*	3
Apple-Grape-Pineapple *(Welch's Orchard)*	3
Apple-Grape-Raspberry *(Welch's Orchard)*	3
Cherry Cider *(R. W. Knudsen)*	★
Citrus Beverage *(Five Alive)*	3
Cranberry Juice Cocktail *(Seneca)*	3
Cranberry Nectar *(R. W. Knudsen)*	★
Cranberry-Apple Juice Cocktail *(Seneca)*	3
Cranberry-Apple Juice Cocktail *(Welch's)*	3
Cranberry-Orange Cocktail *(Welch's)*	3
Cranberry-Raspberry Cocktail *(Welch's)*	3
Fruit Punch *(Minute Maid)*	3
Grape *(Bel-air)*	3
Grape *(Minute Maid)*	3
Grape, Sweetened *(Seneca)*	3
Grape, Sweetened *(Welch's)*	3
Grape, Unsweetened *(Seneca)*	★
Grape, Unsweetened *(Welch's)*	★
Grapefruit *(Citrus Hill)*	★
Grapefruit *(Kraft)*	★
Grapefruit *(Minute Maid)*	★
Harvest Blend *(Welch's Orchard)*	3
Harvest Orchard *(Welch's Orchard)*	3
Lemon *(Minute Maid)*	★
Lemonade *(Bel-air)*	3
Lemonade *(Minute Maid)*	3
Lemonade, Country Style *(Minute Maid)*	3
Mandarin Tangerine, Pure & Light *(Dole)*	★
Mountain Cherry *(Dole)*	★
Natural Apple *(R. W. Knudsen)*	★
Natural Breakfast *(R. W. Knudsen)*	★
North Country Raspberry *(Welch's Orchard)*	3

1 = High Fat 2 = High Sodium 3 = High Refined Sugar 5 = Cholesterol
1+ = Very High Fat 2+ = Very High Sodium 4 = Highly Processed ★= Better Choice

VARIETY *(Brand)*   RATING CODE

Variety (Brand)	Rating Code
Orange *(Bel-air)*	★
Orange *(Citrus Hill)*	★
Orange *(Dole)*	★
Orange *(Donald Duck)*	★
Orange *(Florida Gold)*	★
Orange *(Minute Maid)*	★
Orange *(R. W. Knudsen)*	★
Orange *(Tree Sweet)*	★
Orange *(Tropicana)*	★
Orange Plus Calcium *(Citrus Hill)*	★
Orange Plus Calcium *(Kraft)*	★
Orange Plus Calcium *(Minute Maid)*	★
Orange, Country Style *(Minute Maid)*	★
Orange, Homestyle *(Tropicana)*	★
Orange, Pulp Free *(Minute Maid)*	★
Orange, Reduced Acid *(Minute Maid)*	★
Orchard Peach, Pure & Light *(Dole)*	★
Pineapple *(Dole)*	★
Pineapple-Orange-Banana *(Dole)*	★
Pineapple-Orange-Guava *(Dole)*	★
Pineapple-Passion Fruit-Banana *(Dole)*	★
Pink Grapefruit *(Bel-air)*	★
Pink Lemonade *(Bel-air)*	3
Pink Lemonade *(Minute Maid)*	3
Raspberry Nectar *(R. W. Knudsen)*	★
Raspberry-Cranberry Juice Cocktail *(Seneca)*	3
Tropicals, Guava *(Welch's Orchard)*	3
Tropicals, Passion Fruit *(Welch's Orchard)*	3
Tropicals, Pineapple-Banana *(Welch's Orchard)*	3
REFRIGERATED	
Apple *(Hardin)*	★
Apple *(Mr. Pure)*	★
Apple *(Tree Top)*	★

1 = High Fat	2 = High Sodium	3 = High Refined Sugar	5 = Cholesterol
1+ = Very High Fat	2+ = Very High Sodium	4 = Highly Processed	★= Better Choice

VARIETY *(Brand)*   RATING CODE

Apple *(Veryfine)*	★		
Apple Cider *(Hardin)*	★		
Apple Punch *(Minute Maid)*		3	
Apple, Pure Unsweetened *(Kraft)*	★		
Berry Juicy *(Premium)*	★		
Boysenberry Delight *(Nice & Natural)*	★		
Caribbean Splash *(Chiquita)*	★		
Cherry Delight *(Nice & Natural)*	★		
Citrus Beverage Five Alive *(Five Alive)*		3	
Citrus Punch *(Minute Maid)*		3	
Cranberry Delight *(Nice & Natural)*	★		
Fruit Punch *(Minute Maid)*		3	
Grape *(Mr. Pure)*	★		
Grape *(Veryfine)*	★		
Grape, Pure Unsweetened *(Kraft)*	★		
Grape, Sweetened *(Welch's)*		3	
Grape, Unsweetened *(Welch's)*	★		
Grapeade *(Minute Maid)*		3	
Grapefruit *(Citrus Hill)*	★		
Grapefruit *(Kraft)*	★		
Grapefruit *(Libby's)*	★		
Grapefruit *(Mr. Pure)*	★		
Grapefruit *(Tropicana)*	★		
Grapefruit *(Veryfine)*	★		
Grapefruit Cocktail *(Minute Maid)*		3	
Grapefruit Plus Calcium *(Citrus Hill)*	★		
Grapefruit, Red *(Fresh 'n Natural)*	★		
Grapefruit, Ruby Red *(Squeezins)*	★		
Lemon *(Real Lemon)*	★		
Lemonade *(Minute Maid)*		3	
Lemonade *(Newman's Own)*		3	
Lemonade, Country Style *(Minute Maid)*		3	
Orange *(Bel-air)*	★		

VARIETY *(Brand)*   RATING CODE

Variety (Brand)	Rating
Orange *(Borden)*	★
Orange *(Citrus Hill)*	★
Orange *(Donald Duck)*	★
Orange *(Florida Gold)*	★
Orange *(Florida's Favorite)*	★
Orange *(Fresh 'n Natural)*	★
Orange *(Kraft)*	★
Orange *(Minute Maid)*	★
Orange *(Mr. Pure)*	★
Orange *(Skweezin's)*	★
Orange *(Tropicana)*	★
Orange *(Veryfine)*	★
Orange Plus Calcium *(Citrus Hill)*	★
Orange Plus Calcium *(Minute Maid)*	★
Orange, Country Style *(Minute Maid)*	★
Orange, Homestyle *(Tropicana)*	★
Orange, Pulp Free *(Minute Maid)*	★
Orange-Banana *(Chiquita)*	★
Orange-Pineapple *(Kraft)*	★
Orange-Pineapple *(Tropicana)*	★
Orange-Strawberry-Banana *(Tropicana)*	★
Papaya Delight *(Nice & Natural)*	★
Peach Delight *(Nice & Natural)*	★
Pineapple *(Dole)*	★
Pineapple-Grapefruit *(Tropicana)*	★
Pineapple-Orange *(Dole)*	★
Pineapple-Orange *(Mr. Pure)*	★
Pineapple-Orange-Guava *(Dole)*	★
Pineapple-Passion Fruit-Banana *(Dole)*	★
Pink Lemonade *(Minute Maid)*	3
Red Raspberry Delight *(Nice & Natural)*	★
Tropical Squeeze *(Chiquita)*	★

1 = High Fat	3 = High Refined Sugar	5 = Cholesterol
1+ = Very High Fat	4 = Highly Processed	★= Better Choice
2 = High Sodium		
2+ = Very High Sodium		

MEATS

Most canned meats are of the seafood variety. If you're used to fresh seafood, you won't think much of canned. However, if you live where fresh seafood is not as accessible, you may not know the difference. There are a lot of good choices such as mackerel, salmon, sardines, tuna and so on. We do, however, need to watch for the salt and oil. To remove salt, just rinse for a few seconds under running water and most will be removed. Some varieties are packed in oil and some in water. Choose the water if you're wanting to lower your fat intake. Overall, I rate this group quite good.

Most canned meats are free of additives and preservatives, with the exception of a few varieties such as *Underwood's* Light Deviled Ham, which contains sodium nitrite and hickory smoke, and *Spam*, which has nitrites.

Most all frozen meats are fresh-frozen, and therefore are good choices unless they have been injected with a basting solution such as whole turkeys sometimes are. For example: *Butterball* Turkey is injected with polysorbate 60 and artificial flavor. All fresh-frozen meats have to be cooked, and therefore are not of the quick and easy type. However, there are some very good choices offered here.

Based on research, it is my opinion that many refrigerated meats are very dangerous. Most contain nitrites which are proven to be carcinogenic (cancer causing). These processed meats are easily identified by their pink color. As examples: ham, turkey ham, frankfurters, bologna, salami, etc. As you can see, very few refrigerated meats made *The Food Bible*. However, there are a few good choices such as *Hormel's* Chicken by George and the *Louis Rich* varieties listed below.

VARIETY (Brand)   RATING CODE

MEATS		
CANNED		
Anchovies with Capers (Durkee)	1+ 2+	5
Anchovy Fillets (Durkee)	1 2+	5
Anchovy Fillets (Reese)	1 2+	5
Anchovy Fillets in Olive Oil (Crown-Prince)	1+ 2+	5
Anchovy Paste (Roland)	1 2+	5
Bonito in Oil (Iberia)	1+ 2	5
Chicken, Boned (Sweet Sue)	1 2	5
Chicken, Breast Chunk (Hormel)	1 2	5
Chicken, Breast Chunk, No Salt (Hormel)	1	5
Chicken, Chunk (Hormel)	1 2	5
Chicken, Chunk (Valley Fresh)	1 2	5
Chicken, Mixin (Swanson)	1+ 2	5
Chicken, White (Swanson)	1 2+	5
Chicken, White & Dark (Hormel)	1 2	5
Chicken, White & Dark (Swanson)	1 2	5
Chicken, White (Valley Fresh)	1 2	5
Chicken, Whole (Sweet Sue)	1 2	5
Clam Juice (Bookbinders)	2+	
Clam Juice (Doxsee)	2+	
Clams (Crown Prince)	2+	5
Clams, Chopped (Geisha)	2+	5
Clams, Minced (Gourmet Award)	2+	5
Crab Meat, Claw (Sea Fare)	2+	5
Crab Meat, White (Sea Fare)	2+	5
Cuttle Fish in Olive Oil (Vigo)	1+ 2+	5
Herring in Beer Sauce (Gosch)	1+ 2+	5
Herring in Horseradish Sauce (Gosch)	1+ 2+	5
Herring in Horseradish Sauce (Roland)	1+ 2+	5
Herring in Hot Sauce (Beach Cliff)	1+ 2+	5
Herring in Mustard Sauce (Gosch)	1+ 2+	5
Herring in Mustard Sauce (Roland)	1+ 2+	5
Herring in Soybean Oil (Beach Cliff)	1+ 2	5
Herring in Tangy Mustard (Beach Cliff)	1+ 2+	5

1 = High Fat   2 = High Sodium   3 = High Refined Sugar   5 = Cholesterol
1+ = Very High Fat   2+ = Very High Sodium   4 = Highly Processed   ★= Better Choice

VARIETY *(Brand)*   RATING CODE

Variety (Brand)			
Herring in Tomato Sauce *(Gosch)*	1+	2+	5
Herring in Tomato Sauce *(Roland)*	1+	2+	5
Herring in Wine Sauce *(Roland)*	1+	2	5
Mackerel *(Crown Prince)*	1	2	5
Mackerel *(Geisha)*	1	2	5
Mackerel *(Old South)*	1	2	5
Mackerel *(Star Kist)*	1	2	5
Mackerel *(3-Diamonds)*	1	2	5
Mackerel *(Van Camp's)*	1	2	5
Mackerel *(Wel-Pac)*	1	2	5
Mackerel in Tomato Sauce *(Wel-Pac)*	1	2	5
Mackerel, Kabayaki *(Wel-Pac)*	1	2	5
Mackerel, Skinless, Boneless *(Roland)*	1		5
Mackerel, Teriyaki *(Wel-Pac)*	1	2	5
Mussels in Butter *(Gourmet Award)*	1+	2+	5
Oysters *(Crown Prince)*	1	2	5
Oysters *(Durkee)*	1	2	5
Oysters *(Gourmet Award)*	1	2	5
Oysters *(Orleans)*	1	2	5
Oysters *(3-Diamonds)*	1	2	5
Oysters, Pieces & Whole *(Reese)*	1	2	5
Oysters, Whole *(Geisha)*	1	2	5
Salmon, Blueback *(Season)*	1	2	5
Salmon, Chum *(Honey Boy)*	1	2+	5
Salmon, Keta *(Pink Beauty)*	1	2+	5
Salmon, Keta, Skinless & Boneless *(Chicken of the Sea)*	1	2+	5
Salmon, Pink *(Bandon SeaPack)*	1		5
Salmon, Pink *(Bumble Bee)*	1	2+	5
Salmon, Pink *(Chicken of the Sea)*	1	2+	5
Salmon, Pink *(Deming's)*	1	2+	5
Salmon, Pink *(Featherweight)*	1		5
Salmon, Pink *(Honey Boy)*	1	2+	5
Salmon, Pink *(Hormel)*	1	2+	5

1 = High Fat	2 = High Sodium	3 = High Refined Sugar	5 = Cholesterol
1+ = Very High Fat	2+ = Very High Sodium	4 = Highly Processed	★ = Better Choice

VARIETY *(Brand)*   RATING CODE

Variety (Brand)			
Salmon, Pink *(Libby's)*	1	2+	5
Salmon, Pink *(Pink Beauty)*	1	2+	5
Salmon, Pink *(Royal Pink)*	1	2+	5
Salmon, Pink *(Sea Alaska)*	1	2+	5
Salmon, Pink, Skinless & Boneless *(Chicken of the Sea)*	1	2+	5
Salmon, Red *(Bumble Bee)*	1	2+	5
Salmon, Red *(Honey Boy)*	1	2	5
Salmon, Red *(Royal Red)*	1	2+	5
Salmon, Red Sockeye *(Libby's)*	1	2	5
Salmon, Red Sockeye *(S & W)*	1	2+	5
Salmon, Red Sockeye *(Sea Alaska)*	1	2+	5
Salmon, Silver Bandon *(SeaPack)*	1		5
Salmon, Skinless & Boneless *(Honey Boy)*	1	2+	5
Sardines in Mustard Sauce *(Beach Cliff)*	1+	2+	5
Sardines in Mustard Sauce *(Gourmet Award)*	1+	2+	5
Sardines in Oil *(Crown Prince)*	1+		5
Sardines in Oil *(Neptune)*	1+	2	5
Sardines in Olive Oil *(Fancifood)*	1+	2	5
Sardines in Olive Oil *(Vigo)*	1+	2	5
Sardines in Olive Oil, "Hot" *(Vigo)*	1+	2	5
Sardines in Sardine Oil *(Fancifood)*	1+	2	5
Sardines in Spring Water *(Port Clyde)*	1+	2	5
Sardines in Tomato Sauce *(Crown Prince)*	1+	2	5
Sardines in Tomato Sauce *(Fancifood)*	1+	2	5
Sardines in Tomato Sauce *(Iberia)*	1+	2	5
Sardines in Tomato Sauce *(Polar)*	1+	2	5
Sardines in Tomato Sauce *(Vigo)*	1+	2	5
Sardines in Tomato Sauce *(Wel-Pac)*	1+	2	5
Sardines in Tomato Sauce with Oil *(Gourmet Award)*	1+	2	5
Sardines in Tomato Sauce, No Oil *(Gourmet Award)*	1+	2	5
Sardines, Brisling *(Durkee)*	1+	2	5
Sardines, Brisling *(Reese)*	1+	2+	5
Sardines, Norway, No Salt Added *(Crown Prince)*	1+		5

1 = High Fat 1+ = Very High Fat 2 = High Sodium 2+ = Very High Sodium 3 = High Refined Sugar 4 = Highly Processed 5 = Cholesterol ★= Better Choice

VARIETY *(Brand)*   RATING CODE

Sardines, Skinless & Boneless *(Gourmet Award)*	1+ 2	5
Sardines, Skinless & Boneless in Olive Oil *(Fancifood)*	1+ 2	5
Sardines, Skinless & Boneless in Olive Oil *(Vigo)*	1+ 2	5
Sardines, Skinless & Boneless in Soya, Oil *(Fancifood)*	1+ 2	5
Sardines, Skinless & Boneless in Water, No Salt *(Fancifood)*	1+	5
Shrimp, Deveined *(Marvelous)*		5
TUNA IN OIL		
Tuna, Chunk Light *(Bumble Bee)*	1+ 2	5
Tuna, Chunk Light *(Chicken of the Sea)*	1+ 2	5
Tuna, Chunk Light *(Geisha)*	1+ 2	5
Tuna, Chunk Light *(Star Kist)*	1+ 2	5
Tuna, Chunk Light *(3-Diamonds)*	1+ 2	5
Tuna, Chunk Light, High Protein *(Carnation)*	1+ 2	5
Tuna, Solid White *(Bumble Bee)*	1+ 2	5
Tuna, Solid White *(Chicken of the Sea)*	1+ 2	5
TUNA IN WATER		
Tuna *(Breast Of Chicken)*	2+	5
Tuna *(Deep Sea)*	2+	5
Tuna *(Miramonte)*	2+	5
Tuna *(Season)*	2+	5
Tuna, Chunk Light *(Bumble Bee)*	2+	5
Tuna, Chunk Light *(Carnation)*	2+	5
Tuna, Chunk Light *(Chicken of the Sea)*	2+	5
Tuna, Chunk Light *(Featherweight)*		5
Tuna, Chunk Light *(Sea Trader)*	2+	5
Tuna, Chunk Light *(Star Kist)*	2+	5
Tuna, Chunk Light *(3-Diamonds)*	2+	5
Tuna, Chunk Light *(Weight Watchers)*	2+	5
Tuna, Chunk Light, Diet *(Chicken of the Sea)*		5
Tuna, Chunk Light, Diet *(Star Kist)*		5
Tuna, Chunk Light, 50% Less Salt *(Chicken of the Sea)*	2	5
Tuna, Chunk White *(Bumble Bee)*	2+	5
Tuna, Flake Light *(Rainbow)*	2+	5
Tuna, Lite, Seasoned with Oil *(Chicken of the Sea)*	2+	5

1 = High Fat	2 = High Sodium	3 = High Refined Sugar	5 = Cholesterol
1+ = Very High Fat	2+ = Very High Sodium	4 = Highly Processed	★= Better Choice

VARIETY (Brand)   RATING CODE

Item				
Tuna, No Salt (Miramonte)				5
Tuna, Select, 60% Less Salt (Star Kist)		2		5
Tuna, Solid Light (Star Kist)		2+		5
Tuna, Solid White (Bumble Bee)		2+		5
Tuna, Solid White (Chicken of the Sea)		2+		5
Tuna, Solid White (Geisha)		2+		5
Tuna, Solid White (Sea Trader)		2+		5
Tuna, Solid White (Star Kist)		2+		5
Tuna, Solid White (Weight Watchers)		2+		5
Turkey, White (Swanson)	1	2		5
Turkey, White (Valley Fresh)	1	2		5
FROZEN				
Baby Clams (MACO)				5
Capon with Giblets (Minowa)	1			5
Capon with Giblets (Sleepy Eye)	1			5
Catfish Fillets (Delta Pride)				5
Catfish Fillets (Rupert's)	1			5
Catfish Fillets (Taste O' Sea)	1			5
Chicken (Cookin' Good)	1			5
Chicken Breast, Ground (Cal Golden Farms)				5
Cod Fillets (Booth)				5
Cod Fillets (Firelight)				5
Cod Fillets (Gorton's)				5
Cod Fillets (Taste O' Sea)				5
Cod Fillets (Van de Kamp's)				5
Crab Meat, Snow (Wakefield)		2+		5
Duckling (Concord Crown)	1			5
Duckling (Manor House)	1			5
Duckling (Tyson)	1			5
Flounder Fillets (Booth)				5
Flounder Fillets (Captain's Choice)				5
Flounder Fillets (Fulton's)				5
Flounder Fillets (Galletti Bros.)				5

1 = High Fat   2 = High Sodium   3 = High Refined Sugar   5 = Cholesterol
1+ = Very High Fat   2+ = Very High Sodium   4 = Highly Processed   ★= Better Choice

VARIETY *(Brand)*   RATING CODE

VARIETY (Brand)	1	2	5
Flounder Fillets *(Gorton's)*			5
Flounder Fillets *(Sea Pack)*			5
Flounder Fillets *(Taste O' Sea)*			5
Flounder Fillets *(Van de Kamp's)*			5
Goose *(Oak Valley Farms)*	1		5
Goose *(Sleepy Eye)*	1		5
Goose *(Whetstone Valley)*	1		5
Grouper Fillets *(Fulton's)*			5
Haddock *(Captain's Choice)*			5
Haddock *(Taste O' Sea)*			5
Haddock Fillets *(Booth)*			5
Haddock Fillets *(Taste O' Sea)*			5
Halibut *(Captain's Choice)*			5
Hen, Rock Cornish *(Patti jean)*			5
Hen, Rock Cornish *(Tyson)*			5
Hen, Rock Cornish *(Young 'n Tender)*			5
Ocean Perch Fillets *(Taste O' Sea)*			5
Perch *(Captain's Choice)*			5
Perch *(Taste O' Sea)*			5
Perch *(Van de Kamp's)*			5
Pollock Fillets *(Fulton's)*			5
Pollock Fillets *(Taste O' Sea)*			5
Quail *(Manchester Farms)*			5
Quail *(Plantation Quail)*			5
Rabbit *(Nature's Pride)*	1		5
Salmon *(Sea Pack)*			5
Scallops *(Fulton's)*		2	5
Shrimp *(Sau Sea)*			5
Shrimp *(Singleton)*			5
Sole *(Captain's Choice)*			5
Sole *(Taste O' Sea)*			5
Sole *(Van de Kamp's)*			5
Sole Fillets *(Fulton's)*			5

1 = High Fat	2 = High Sodium	3 = High Refined Sugar	5 = Cholesterol
1+ = Very High Fat	2+ = Very High Sodium	4 = Highly Processed	★= Better Choice

VARIETY (Brand)   RATING CODE

Variety (Brand)	Fat	Sodium	Cholesterol
Swordfish (Captain's Choice)			5
Swordfish (Sea Pack)			5
Tuna (Sea Pack)	1		5
Turbot (Taste O' Sea)	2		5
Turkey (Empire)			5
Turkey (Manor House)			5
Turkey (Marval)	1		5
Turkey Breast (Louis Rich)	1		5
Turkey Wings (Louis Rich)	1		5
Turkey, Ground (Louis Rich)	1+		5
Turkey, Ground (Mr. Turkey)	1+		5
Turkey, Ground (Norbest)	1+		5
Turkey, Ground (Shenandoah)	1+		5
Turkey, Ground (Swift Premium)	1+		5
Turkey, Ground, Golden Star (Armour)	1+		5
Turkey, Natural (Carolina Turkey)	1		5
Veal, Ground (Plume De Veau)	1+		5
Whitefish (Fulton's)	1		5
Whiting (Taste O' Sea)			5
Whiting Fillets (Starboard Brand)			5
Whiting Fillets (Taste O' Sea)			5
REFRIGERATED			
Bologna, Chicken (Health Valley)	1+	2+	
Bologna, Turkey (Shelton's)	1+	2+	
Chicken Breast, Oven Roasted, Deli Thin Slices, 96% Fat Free (Louis Rich)		2+	
Chicken Breast, Oven Roasted, Slices 96% Fat Free (Louis Rich)		2+	
Chicken By George, Cajun Style (Hormel)	1	2	5
Chicken By George, Country Mustard & Dill (Hormel)	1	2	5
Chicken By George, Italian Bleu Cheese (Hormel)	1	2+	5
Chicken By George, Lemon Herb (Hormel)		2+	5
Chicken By George, Mexican Style (Hormel)	1	2	5
Chicken By George, Teriyaki (Hormel)		2	5
Chicken By George, Tomato Herb (Hormel)	1	2	5
Chicken, Oven Roasted, White Slices, 93% Fat Free (Louis Rich)		2+	5

VARIETY *(Brand)*   RATING CODE

Franks, Tofu Pups *(Light Life)*	1+ 2	
Franks, Turkey *(Shelton's)*	1+	5
Turkey Breast, Honey Roasted, Slices, 97% Fat Free *(Louis Rich)*	2+	
Turkey Breast, Oven Roasted, Chunk, 95% Fat Free *(Louis Rich)*	2+	
Turkey Breast, Oven Roasted, Chunk *(Mr. Turkey)*	2+	
Turkey Breast, Oven Roasted, Deli Thin Slices, 97% Fat Free *(Louis Rich)*	2+	
Turkey Breast, Oven Roasted, Slices *(Hillshire Farm)*	2+	
Turkey Breast, Oven Roasted, Slices, 97% Fat Free *(Louis Rich)*	2+	
Turkey Breast, Oven Roasted, Slices *(Mr. Turkey)*	2+	
Wieners, Chicken *(Health Valley)*	1+	5
Wieners, Turkey *(Health Valley)*	1+	5

1 = High Fat   2 = High Sodium   3 = High Refined Sugar   5 = Cholesterol
1+ = Very High Fat   2+ = Very High Sodium   4 = Highly Processed   ★= Better Choice

MEXICAN FOODS

Personally, I like the spice and zip of Mexican food, but, as a whole, I cannot rate this group very high. A few products such as *Old El Paso* refried beans contain lard, and *Aztech* flour tortillas contain potassium sorbate and sodium propionate — and they didn't make the *The Food Bible*.

Of the products that did, fat and salt are the big culprits. Products such as tortilla chips, taco shells and tamales are high in fat as well as sodium, and most salsas are high in sodium. Be selective and you'll find some good choices. For example: soft corn tortillas are always better than tortilla chips.

VARIETY *(Brand)*   RATING CODE

MEXICAN FOODS		
Bean Dip, Jalapeño *(Casa Fiesta)*	2+	
Black Beans, Instant Mix *(Fantastic Foods)*	2	
Chapati, Whole Wheat *(Garden of Eatin')*	★	
Chili Beans *(Ashley's)*	2+	
Chili Beans *(Casa Fiesta)*	2+	
Chili Beans *(Ellis)*	2+	
Chili Beans *(Town House)*	2+	
Chili Beans in Sauce *(Chili Man)*	2	
Chili Beans in Sauce, Jalapeño Style *(Chili Man)*	2	
Chili Fixin's, Homestyle, Mild & Regular *(Wolf)*	2+	
Chili Fixin's, Manwich *(Hunt's)*	2+	
Chili Mix, Vegetarian *(Fantastic Foods)*	2	
Chili Mix, Vegetarian with Beans *(Fantastic Foods)*	2	
Chili Peppers, Diced Green *(Zapata)*	2+	
Chili Sauce *(Bennett's)*	2+ 3	
Chili Sauce *(Heinz)*	2+ 3	
Chili Sauce, Red Hot *(Ashley's)*	2+	
Chili Seasoning Mix *(Carroll Shelby's)*	2+	
Chili Seasoning Mix *(Lawry's)*	2+	
Chili Seasoning Mix *(Williams)*	★	
Chili Seasoning Mix with Onions *(Williams)*	★	
Chili Seasoning, No Salt *(La Preferida)*	★	
Chili with Beans *(Gebhardt)*	1+ 2+	5
Chili with Beans *(Rainbow)*	1+ 2+	5
Chili with Beans *(Wolf)*	1+ 2+	5
Chili with Beans, Country *(Stagg)*	1 2+	5
Chili with Beans, Laredo *(Stagg)*	1 2+	5
Chili with Chicken, Spicy *(Hain)*	2+	5
Chili without Beans *(Gebhardt)*	1+ 2	5
Chili without Beans *(Wolf)*	1+ 2	5
Chili, Chicken, Low Sodium *(Shelton's)*	★	
Chili, Chicken, Mild *(Shelton's)*	2+	
Chili, Chicken, Spicy *(Shelton's)*	2+	

1 = High Fat	2 = High Sodium	3 = High Refined Sugar	5 = Cholesterol
1+ = Very High Fat	2+ = Very High Sodium	4 = Highly Processed	★= Better Choice

VARIETY (Brand)
RATING CODE

Variety (Brand)			
Chili, Chicken with Beans (Stagg)	1	2+	5
Chili, Chicken with Beans, Lite (Dennison's)		2	
Chili, Jalapeño with Beans (Wolf)	1+	2+	5
Chili, Jalapeño without Beans (Wolf)	1+	2	5
Chili, Mild Vegetarian with Beans (Health Valley)		2+	
Chili, Mild Vegetarian with Lentils (Health Valley)		2	
Chili, Mild Vegetarian with Beans, No Salt (Health Valley)	★		
Chili, Mild Vegetarian with Lentils, No Salt (Health Valley)	★		
Chili, Spicy Tempeh (Hain)		2+	
Chili, Spicy Vegetarian (Hain)		2+	
Chili, Spicy Vegetarian with Beans (Health Valley)		2+	
Chili, Spicy Vegetarian, Reduced Sodium (Hain)	★		
Chili, Spicy Vegetarian with Beans, No Salt (Health Valley)	★		
Chili, Turkey, Low Sodium (Shelton's)	★		
Chili, Turkey, Mild (Shelton's)		2+	
Chili, Turkey, Spicy (Shelton's)		2+	
Chilpotle Peppers (Del Monte)		2+	
Chipotle Peppers, Pickled (Embasa)		2+	
Corntillas (Garden of Eatin')	★		
Dip, Medium Jalapeño Bean (Hain)		2+	
Dip, Mexican Bean (Hain)		2+	
Dip, Onion Bean (Hain)		2+	
Dip, Taco (Casa Fiesta)		2	
Dip, Taco & Sauce (Hain)		2+	
Enchilada Sauce, Mild & Hot (Ashley's)		2+	
Enchilada Sauce, Mild & Medium (MP)		2+	
Enchiladas, Cheese - [Frozen] (Café Mexico)	1	2+	
Fajita Seasoning Mix (Casa Fiesta)		2+	
Garbanzos (Casa Fiesta)		2+	
Green Chiles, Diced & Whole (La Preferida)		2+	
Green Chili Peppers (Ashley's)		2+	
Green Chilies (Casa Fiesta)		2+	
Green Chilies (Ortega)		2	

1 = High Fat   2 = High Sodium   3 = High Refined Sugar   5 = Cholesterol
1+ = Very High Fat   2+ = Very High Sodium   4 = Highly Processed   ★ = Better Choice

VARIETY *(Brand)*   RATING CODE

Green Chilies, Chopped & Diced *(MP)*	2+		
Green Chilies, Whole & Chopped *(Old El Paso)*	2+		
Hominy, Mexican Style *(Juanita's)*	2+		
Honey-Cins *(el Rio)*	1	3	4
Hot Sauce, Mexi *(Zapata)*	2+		
Hot Sauce, Tennessee Sunshine *(Try Me)*	2+		
Jalapeño Peppers *(Cosmic)*	2+		
Jalapeño Peppers *(Goya)*	2+		
Jalapeño Peppers, Mild Pickled *(Clemente Jacques)*	2+		
Jalapeño Peppers, Nacho Slices *(Clemente Jacques)*	2+		
Jalapeño Peppers, Pickled *(Clemente Jacques)*	2+		
Jalapeño Peppers, Pickled *(Embasa)*	2+		
Jalapeño Relish *(Old El Paso)*	2+		
Jalapeño Sauce *(El Pato)*	2+		
Jalapeños *(Ashley's)*	2+		
Jalapeños, Hot Nacho *(Zapata)*	2+		
Jalapeños, Pickled *(Faraon)*	2+		
Jalapeños, Sliced *(La Victoria)*	2+		
Jalapeños, Whole & Mild Strips *(Zapata)*	2+		
Louisiana Hot Sauce *(La Preferida)*	2		
Mexe-beans *(Old El Paso)*	2+		
Mexican Crisps *(Old El Paso)*	1+	3	4
Mexican Dip, Mild, Medium & Hot *(Jo Anna's)*	2+		
Mexican Rice, Cheese & Mild Green Chilies *(Tio Sancho)*	2+		4
Mexican Rice, Restaurant Style *(Tio Sancho)*	2+		4
Mexican Sauce *(Faraon)*	2+		
Mexican Sauce, Green *(Embasa)*	2+		
Mexican Sauce, Green & Red Home Style *(Embasa)*	2+		
Mexican Sauce, Home Style *(Embasa)*	2+		
Nachips *(Old El Paso)*	1		
Nacho Chips, No Salt *(La Preferida)*	1+		
Peppers, Roasted Red Bell *(Mezzetta)*	2+		
Picante Sauce, Mild, Medium & Hot *(Old El Paso)*	2+		

VARIETY *(Brand)*   RATING CODE

Picante Sauce, Mild, Medium & Hot *(Pace)*	2+
Picante Sauce, Chunky, Mild & Medium *(Rosarita)*	2+
Picante Sauce, Mild & Medium *(MP)*	2+
Pilaf Mix, Spanish Brown Rice *(Fantastic Foods)*	2+
Pinto Beans *(Casa Fiesta)*	2+
Pinto Beans *(Old El Paso)*	2+
Refried Beans *(Little Bear)*	2
Refried Beans *(Tio Sancho)*	2+
Refried Beans *(Zapata)*	2+
Refried Beans, Instant Mix *(Fantastic Foods)*	2
Refried Beans, Spicy *(Little Bear)*	2
Refried Beans, Spicy *(Zapata)*	2+
Refried Beans, Vegetarian *(Old El Paso)*	2+
Salsa Casera *(Herdez)*	2+
Salsa, Chunky *(Frito Lay)*	2+
Salsa, Chunky, Hot, Medium & Mild *(Tio Sancho)*	2+
Salsa, Green Chili *(Santa Rosa Salsa)*	2+
Salsa, Green Chili, Medium & Mild *(Territorial House)*	2+
Salsa, Hot & Mild *(Hain)*	2+
Salsa, Chunky, Medium *(Frito Lay)*	2+
Salsa, Chunky Dip, Medium *(Mission)*	2+
Salsa, Thick'n'Chunky, Mild, Medium & Hot *(Old El Paso)*	2+
Salsa, Thick'n'Chunky, Mild, Medium & Hot *(Pace)*	2+
Serrano Peppers, Pickled *(Faraon)*	2+
Spanish Rice *(Old El Paso)*	2+ 4
Taco Dip *(Ashley's)*	2
Taco Sauce *(Cattlebaron)*	2+
Taco Sauce *(Old El Paso)*	2+
Taco Sauce, Medium *(Old El Paso)*	2+
Taco Sauce, Mild *(Chi-Chi's)*	2+ 3
Taco Seasoning *(el Rio)*	2+
Taco Shells *(el Rio)*	1
Taco Shells *(Little Bear)*	1 2

VARIETY *(Brand)*   RATING CODE

Taco Shells *(Old El Paso)*	1
Taco Shells, Blue *(Little Bear)*	1
Taco Shells, Mini *(Old El Paso)*	1+

Taco Shells, Super Size *(Old El Paso)*	1+	
Tamales with Chili Gravy *(Old El Paso)*	1+ 2	5
Tamales, Beef *(Ashley's)*	1+ 2	5

Tamales, Blue Corn with Chicken [Frozen] *(Col. Sanchez)*	1	5
Tamales, Green Chili with Cheese [Frozen] *(Col. Sanchez)*	1+	5
Tamales, Red Chili with Tofu [Frozen] *(Col. Sanchez)*	1+ 2	

Tomatoes & Green Chiles *(Ashley's)*	2+
Tomatoes & Green Chilies *(Old El Paso)*	2+
Tortilla Chips *(Chi-Chi's)*	1+

Tortilla Chips, Cantina Style *(Frito Lay)*	1+
Tortilla Chips, Restaurant Style *(Frito Lay)*	1+
Tortilla Chips, Sesame *(Hain)*	1

Tortilla Chips, Sesame, No Salt *(Hain)*	1
Tortilla Chips, Sesame Cheese *(Hain)*	1 2
Tortillas, Blue Corn *(Garden of Eatin')*	★

Tortillas, Soft Corn *(Casa del Pueblo)*	★
Tortillas, Soft Corn *(Del Sol)*	★
Tortillas, Soft Corn *(El Pato)*	★

Tortillas, Soft Corn *(Piñata)*	★
Tortillas, Soft Corn *(Jimenez)*	★
Tortillas, Soft Corn *(El Muchacho)*	★

Tortillas, Soft Corn *(Our House)*	★
Tortillas, Sprouted Wheat *(Alvarado St. Bakery)*	★
Tortillas, Whole Wheat *(Garden of Eatin')*	★

Tostaco Shells *(Old El Paso)*	1
Tostada Shells *(el Rio)*	1
Tostada Shells *(Little Bear)*	1 2

Tostada Shells *(Old El Paso)*	1
Tostada Shells, Blue Corn *(Little Bear)*	1 2

MILK

Practically all brands of milk are local; so very few ratings are offered by brands. I consider any milk over 1% to be high in fat; so the skim, 1/2 % and 1% are our best choices. I have had a number of clients state that they cannot stand the taste of 1% milk when they are used to whole milk. I have found that a gradual switch is more comfortable. At first, try mixing whole milk in equal portions with 1%, then as you become used to that taste, decrease the whole milk gradually until you're drinking only 1% milk. This same process can get you on down to skim milk, if so desired. I'll assure you that once you've made the switch, you will not be able to "stomach" whole milk.

Most all canned and powdered milks are free of additives and preservatives; however, there is a great deal of difference in the fat and sugar content of the canned milks. Evaporated skimmed milk is the best choice and is excellent to use as a coffee creamer as well as in cooking. Nonfat dry milk is an excellent low-cost choice for cereals and baking as well as drinking.

All forms of cream are very high in fat; however, there is some good news. Let's compare:

ITEM	AMOUNT	CALORIES	GRAMS OF FAT	% OF FAT
Half & Half	1 TB	20	1.8 g.	81%
Sour Cream	1 TB	26	2.5 g.	87%
Whipping Cream	1 TB	52	5.6 g.	97%
Butter	1 TB	108	12.0 g.	100%

Now for the good news! Since it is so easy to use a tablespoon of butter on a baked potato, next time, try only sour cream and see if that will work for you. By doing this, you have certainly lowered your fat consumption. *Two level tablespoons* of sour cream have about the same grams of fat as *one level teaspoon* of butter.

I rate the creams above butter, but that's about it. For optimum health, both really need to be limited in our daily diets.

VARIETY *(Brand)*   RATING CODE

MILK
CANNED

Variety (Brand)	1	2	3	5
Evaporated Milk, 2% *(Carnation)*	★			
Evaporated Milk, Goat *(Meyenberg)*	1			
Evaporated Milk, Skimmed *(Carnation)*	★			
Evaporated Milk, Skimmed *(Pet)*	★			
Evaporated Milk, Whole *(Carnation)*	1+			
Evaporated Milk, Whole *(Lucerne)*	1+			
Evaporated Milk, Whole *(Milnot)*	1+			
Evaporated Milk, Whole *(Pet)*	1+			
Evaporated Filled Milk, Dairymate *(Pet)*	1			
Evaporated Sweetened, Eagle Brand *(Borden)*			3	
Evaporated Sweetened Condensed Milk *(Carnation)*			3	
Evaporated Sweetened, Dairy Sweet *(Milnot)*			3	
Filled Milk *(Rainbow)*	1			
CREAMS				
Half & Half *(Borden)*	1+			
Half & Half *(Lucerne)*	1+			
Sour Cream *(Alta•Dena)*	1+			
Sour Cream *(Borden)*	1+			
Sour Cream *(Breakstone's)*	1+			
Sour Cream *(Carnation)*	1+			
Sour Cream *(Daisy)*	1+			
Sour Cream *(Lucerne)*	1+			
Sour Cream & Chives *(Lucerne)*	1+			
Sour Cream, Light *(Daisy)*	1+			
Sour Cream, Light *(Lucerne)*	1+			
Sour Cream, Light Choice *(Breakstone's)*	1+			
Whipping Cream *(Lucerne)*	1+			5
Whipping Cream, Heavy *(Dairy Pure)*	1+			5
DRY				
Dry Milk, Nonfat *(Carnation)*		2		
Dry Milk, Nonfat *(Lucerne)*		2		
Dry Milk, Nonfat *(Sanalac)*		2		

1 = High Fat   2 = High Sodium   3 = High Refined Sugar   5 = Cholesterol
1+ = Very High Fat   2+ = Very High Sodium   4 = Highly Processed   ★= Better Choice

VARIETY *(Brand)*   RATING CODE

VARIETY (Brand)	★	1	2	5
REFRIGERATED				
Milk, Skim *(Lucerne)*	★			
Milk, Skim *(Schepps)*			2	
Milk, Skim *(Weight Watchers)*			2	
Milk, Skim, Lite Line *(Borden)*	★			
Acidophilus, 1 1/2% *(Borden)*		1		
Acidophilus, 2% *(Lucerne)*		1		
Acidophilus, Lowfat *(Alta·Dena)*		1		
Buttermilk *(Alta·Dena)*	★			
Buttermilk, 1 1/2% *(Lucerne)*			2	
Chocolate Milk, Lowfat *(Alta·Dena)*	★			
Goat Milk *(Meyenberg)*		1		
Kefir, Boysenberry *(Kefir)*		1		5
Kefir, Peach *(Kefir)*		1		5
Kefir, Pineapple *(Kefir)*		1		5
Kefir, Red Raspberry *(Kefir)*		1		5
Kefir, Strawberry *(Kefir)*		1		5
Milk, 1% *(Lucerne)*	★			
Milk, 1/2% *(Lucerne)*	★			
Milk, 2% *(Lucerne)*		1		
Milk, 2% Hi-Protein *(Borden)*		1		
Milk, Lactose Reduced *(Lactaid)*	★			
Milk, Whole *(Alta·Dena)*		1+		5
Milk, Whole *(Borden)*		1+		5
Milk, Whole *(Lucerne)*		1+		5
Milk, Whole *(Schepps)*		1+		5

1 = High Fat   2 = High Sodium   3 = High Refined Sugar   5 = Cholesterol
1+ = Very High Fat   2+ = Very High Sodium   4 = Highly Processed   ★= Better Choice

NUTS AND SEEDS

I really like nuts and seeds, and I frequently add them to pancakes, muffins, salads, casseroles, etc. They all are very high in fat but also very nutritious. In fact, I even rate almonds as a superfood — very, very nutritious. If I had to pick one source for us to receive our required fat, I would pick nuts and seeds.

When they are available (generally in season), the fresh raw nuts and seeds are the best choices. Canning and long shelf life can destroy some nutrients. Some packaged nuts such as *Planters* peanuts contain additives such as MSG and cottonseed oil, and red pistachio nuts contain artificial color. As a group though, I rate them high — with limited consumption.

VARIETY *(Brand)*   RATING CODE

NUTS AND SEEDS		
NUTS		
Almonds, Blanched *(Blue Diamond)*	1+	
Almonds, Blanched & Slivered *(Azar)*	1+	
Almonds, Honey Roasted *(Blue Diamond)*	1+	3
Almonds, Onion Garlic *(Blue Diamond)*	1+	
Almonds, Salted *(Blue Diamond)*	1+	
Almonds, Sliced *(Dole)*	1+	
Almonds, Whole Natural *(Blue Diamond)*	1+	
Almonds, Whole Sliced *(Planters)*	1+	
Cashew & Peanut Mix *(Eagle)*	1+	3
Cashew Halves *(Fisher)*	1+	
Cashews, Honey Roast *(Eagle)*	1+	3
Cashews, Lightly Salted *(Eagle)*	1+	
Corn Kernels, Roasted & Salted *(Nut House)*	1+ 2	
Mixed Nuts *(Azar)*	1+	
Mixed Nuts *(Eagle)*	1+	
Nut Topping *(Planters)*	1+	
Peanut Candy *(Planters)*	1+	3
Peanut Topping *(Azar)*	1+	
Peanuts, Cinnamon Roast *(Eagle)*	1+	3
Peanuts, Dry Roasted *(Fisher)*	1+	
Peanuts, Dry Roasted, Unsalted *(Fisher)*	1+	
Peanuts, Dry Roasted, Unsalted *(Planters)*	1+	
Peanuts, Honey Dry Roasted *(Planters)*	1+	3
Peanuts, Honey Roasted *(Eagle)*	1+	3
Peanuts, Honey Roasted *(Fisher)*	1+	3
Peanuts, In Shell & Salted *(Fisher)*	1+ 2	
Peanuts, In Shell & Salted *(Nut House)*	1+ 2	
Peanuts, In Shell & Unsalted *(Fisher)*	1+	
Peanuts, Lightly Salted *(Eagle)*	1+	
Peanuts, Lightly Salted *(Planters)*	1+	
Peanuts, Maple Roast *(Eagle)*	1+	3
Peanuts, Party *(Fisher)*	1+	
Peanuts, Raw *(Ellis)*	1+	

1 = High Fat	2 = High Sodium	3 = High Refined Sugar	5 = Cholesterol
1+ = Very High Fat	2+ = Very High Sodium	4 = Highly Processed	★= Better Choice

VARIETY (Brand)   RATING CODE

Peanuts, Raw Spanish (Azar)	1+
Peanuts, Roasted (Nut House)	1+
Peanuts, Spanish (Fisher)	1+
Peanuts, Spanish, Lightly Salted (Fisher)	1+
Peanuts, Sweet 'N Crunchy (Planters)	1+ 3
Pecan Halves (Planters)	1+
Pecan Halves & Pieces (Party Pride)	1+
Pecan Pieces (Ellis)	1+
Pecan Pieces & Whole (Azar)	1+
Pecans (Del Cerro)	1+
Pistachios, Dry Roasted, Plain (Blue Diamond)	1+
Pistachios, Regular Dry Roasted (Planters)	1+ 2
Raw Nuts, Not Roasted or Salted (Azar)	1+
Raw Nuts, Not Roasted or Salted (Evon's)	1+
Raw Nuts, Not Roasted or Salted (Laura Scudder's)	1+
Walnuts, English (Azar)	1+
Walnuts, English (Ellis)	1+

SEEDS

Pumpkin Seeds (Nut House)	1+ 2
Sesame, Hulled (Arrowhead Mills)	1+
Sesame, Whole (Arrowhead Mills)	1+
Sesame, Whole (Stone-Buhr)	1+
Sunflower Kernels, Roasted & Salted (David)	1+
Sunflower Seeds in Shell (Guys)	1+
Sunflower Seeds in Shell (Planters)	1+
Sunflower Seeds, Roasted & Salted in Shell (Good Sense)	1+
Sunflower Seeds, Toasted & Salted in Shell (Azar)	1+
Sunflower, Hulled (Stone-Buhr)	1+
Sunflower, Hulled & Dry Roasted (Fisher)	1+
Sunflower, Whole (Arrowhead Mills)	1+

1 = High Fat	2 = High Sodium	3 = High Refined Sugar	5 = Cholesterol
1+ = Very High Fat	2+ = Very High Sodium	4 = Highly Processed	★= Better Choice

OILS

Oils are a very highly processed item that is 100% fat. We receive lots of fat, lots of calories, and some vitamin E from oils. Since I know that we are going to use oil, let's choose the best. In my opinion, safflower is the best choice followed by canola, sunflower, corn and soybean oils. These are the least saturated and the lowest in monounsaturated fats — which I favor.

The key, though, is to limit all oils as much as possible. CAUTION: Even though some bottles say "no cholesterol," they are still 100% fat. I see many people switching from animal fat to vegetable fat, and they think they're on a health kick. Whether you're standing in the middle of the fire or on the edge of the fire, you're still going to get burned. In other words, limit all fat consumption.

VARIETY *(Brand)*   RATING CODE

OILS		
All Blend *(Hain)*	1+	4
Almond *(Hain)*	1+	4
Almond *(Spectrum Naturals)*	1+	4
Apricot Kernel *(Hain)*	1+	4
Avocado *(Hain)*	1+	4
Avocado *(Prepared)*	1+	4
Canola *(Country Pure)*	1+	4
Canola *(Hain)*	1+	4
Canola *(Heart Beat)*	1+	4
Canola *(Loriva)*	1+	4
Canola *(Puritan)*	1+	4
Canola *(Spectrum Naturals)*	1+	4
Corn *(Arrowhead Mills)*	1+	4
Corn *(BestYet)*	1+	4
Corn *(Crisco)*	1+	4
Corn *(Hain)*	1+	4
Corn *(Mazzola)*	1+	4
Corn *(Nu Made)*	1+	4
Corn *(Rainbow)*	1+	4
Corn *(Spectrum Naturals)*	1+	4
Corn *(Wesson)*	1+	4
Grape Seed *(Bonavita)*	1+	4
Grape Seed *(Soleillon)*	1+	4
Grape Seed *(St. Augustine)*	1+	4
Hot Oil *(China Bowl)*	1+	4
Olive *(Arrowhead Mills)*	1+	4
Olive *(Bella)*	1+	4
Olive *(Bertolli)*	1+	4
Olive *(Colavita)*	1+	4
Olive *(Da Vinci)*	1+	4
Olive *(Fillippo Berio)*	1+	4
Olive *(Hain)*	1+	4
Olive *(New Morning)*	1+	4

1 = High Fat   2 = High Sodium   3 = High Refined Sugar   5 = Cholesterol
1+ = Very High Fat   2+ = Very High Sodium   4 = Highly Processed   ★= Better Choice

VARIETY (Brand)   RATING CODE

Olive *(OLIO SASSO)*	1+	4
Olive *(Progresso)*	1+	4
Olive *(Vigo)*	1+	4
Olive, Extra Light *(Pompeian)*	1+	4
Olive, Extra Virgin *(Bella)*	1+	4
Olive, Extra Virgin *(Bertolli)*	1+	4
Olive, Extra Virgin *(Colavita)*	1+	4
Olive, Extra Virgin *(Old Monk)*	1+	4
Olive, Extra Virgin *(Pompeian)*	1+	4
Olive, Italian, Extra Virgin *(Alessi)*	1+	4
Olive, Pepperolio *(Colavita)*	1+	4
Peanut Oil *(Chun King)*	1+	4
Peanut Oil *(Hain)*	1+	4
Peanut Oil *(Hollywood)*	1+	4
Peanut Oil *(Loriva)*	1+	4
Peanut Oil *(Planters)*	1+	4
Peanut Oil *(Spectrum Naturals)*	1+	4
Rice Bran *(Select Origins)*	1+	4
Safflower *(Arrowhead Mills)*	1+	4
Safflower *(Hain)*	1+	4
Safflower *(Hollywood)*	1+	4
Safflower *(Loriva)*	1+	4
Safflower *(Spectrum Naturals)*	1+	4
Safflower, Hi-Oleic *(Hain)*	1+	4
Sesame *(Arrowhead Mills)*	1+	4
Sesame *(China Bowl)*	1+	4
Sesame *(Dynasty)*	1+	4
Sesame *(Hain)*	1+	4
Sesame *(Loriva)*	1+	4
Sesame *(Spectrum Naturals)*	1+	4
Sesame, Toasted *(Arrowhead Mills)*	1+	4
Soy *(Hain)*	1+	4
Soybean, Pure Vegetable *(Mrs. Tuckers)*	1+	4

1 = High Fat   2 = High Sodium   3 = High Refined Sugar   5 = Cholesterol
1+ = Very High Fat   2+ = Very High Sodium   4 = Highly Processed   ★= Better Choice

VARIETY *(Brand)*   RATING CODE

Variety (Brand)		
Soybean, Salad Oil *(Rainbow)*	1+	4
Soybean, Vegetable *(BestYet)*	1+	4
Soybean, Vegetable *(Crisco)*	1+	4
Soybean, Vegetable *(Wesson)*	1+	4
Spray Oil *(Pam)*	1+	4
Spray Oil, Butter Flavor *(Pam)*	1+	4
Sunflower *(Hain)*	1+	4
Sunflower *(Hollywood)*	1+	4
Sunflower *(Loriva)*	1+	4
Sunflower *(Nu Made)*	1+	4
Sunflower *(Spectrum Naturals)*	1+	4
Sunflower *(Wesson)*	1+	4
Walnut *(Hain)*	1+	4
Walnut *(Loriva)*	1+	4
Walnut *(Spectrum Naturals)*	1+	4

1 = High Fat   2 = High Sodium   3 = High Refined Sugar   5 = Cholesterol
1+ = Very High Fat   2+ = Very High Sodium   4 = Highly Processed   ★= Better Choice

ORIENTAL FOODS

I certainly do like Oriental food, particularly stir-fry dishes. I'm especially fond of rice (brown rice) with a variety of vegetables and just a bit of meat. Food preparation has as much to do with Oriental food as the food itself. Very little fat is used in authentic stir-fry, and the minimal cooking that is used to stir-fry is the key. I also like to add tofu to dishes, not so much for its taste, but for its nutritional value.

Most all processed Oriental meals contain MSG and are not in *The Food Bible*. However, my choice is to buy my own vegetables and meat, then add an Oriental spice from *The Food Bible*. This way I can have an Oriental meal without MSG or other additives and preservatives.

VARIETY *(Brand)*   RATING CODE

ORIENTAL FOODS				
Bamboo Shoots *(China Boy)*	★			
Bamboo Shoots *(Chun King)*	★			
Bamboo Shoots *(Dynasty)*	★			
Bamboo Shoots *(Gourmet Award)*	★			
Bamboo Shoots *(Green Giant)*	★			
Bamboo Shoots *(La Choy)*	★			
Bamboo Shoots *(Reese)*	★			
Bean Sprouts *(Chun King)*	★			
Bean Sprouts *(Green Giant)*	★			
Bean Sprouts *(La Choy)*	★			
Bean Sprouts *(Ty Ling)*	★			
Beef & Broccoli, Seasoning Mix *(S & B)*		2+		
Brown Rice Snaps, No Salt, Sesame *(Edward & Sons)*	★			
Brown Rice Snaps, Onion Garlic *(Edward & Sons)*	★			
Brown Rice Snaps, Tamari Sesame *(Edward & Sons)*	★			
Brown Rice Snaps, Zesty Parmesan *(Edward & Sons)*	★			
Chicken Salad, Chinese Seasoning Mix *(S & B)*		2+	3	
Chop Suey Seasoning Mix *(S & B)*		2+		
Chow Mein Seasoning Mix *(S & B)*		2+		
Chow Mein, Mandarin Tofu Classics, No Butter *(Fantastic Foods)*	1	2+		
Cooking Wine *(China Bowl)*		2+		
Corn, Stir-Fry *(KA-ME)*		2		
Crackers, Cheese *(KA-ME)*		2		4
Crackers, Plain *(KA-ME)*				4
Creamy Stroganoff, Tofu Classics, Prepared, No Butter *(Fantastic Foods)*		2		
Egg Rolls, Chicken - [Frozen] *(Lana's)*		2		
Egg Rolls, Pork - [Frozen] *(Lana's)*		2		
Egg Rolls, Shrimp - [Frozen] *(Lana's)*		2		
Egg Rolls, Vegetable - [Frozen] *(Lana's)*		2		
Fish Sauce *(China Bowl)*		2+		
Five Spices *(China King)*	★			
Five Spices *(Dynasty)*	★			
Hot Oil *(China Bowl)*	1+			4

VARIETY (Brand)   RATING CODE

Item	★	1 / 1+	2 / 2+	3	4
Kim Chee *(Frieda)*			2+		
Lemon Chicken Fry, Seasoning Mix *(S & B)*			2+		
Miso Soup, Hearty Red, Instant *(Westbrae)*			2+		
Miso Soup, Mellow White, Instant *(Westbrae)*			2+		
Mushrooms, Enoki *(Green Giant)*			2+		
Mushrooms, Shiitake *(Green Giant)*			2+		
Mustard, Hot *(Port Arthur)*		1+	2+		
Mustard, Hot *(Ty Ling)*			2+		
Noodles, Cellophane *(China Bowl)*	★				
Noodles, Chinese *(China Bowl)*		1	2		4
Noodles, Chow Mein *(China Boy)*		1	2		4
Noodles, Chow Mein *(Chun King)*		1	2		4
Noodles, Rice *(China Boy)*		1	2		4
Pasta Salad, Spicy Oriental, Prepared *(Fantastic Foods)*		1+			
Pea Pods - [Frozen] *(Chun King)*	★				
Pea Pods - [Frozen] *(La Choy)*	★				
Pine Nuts, Chinese *(China Bowl)*		1+			
Plum Sauce *(China Bowl)*				3	
Plum Sauce *(KA-ME)*				3	
Rice Sticks *(China Bowl)*					4
Rice Vinegar *(Nakano)*	★				
Sesame Oil *(China Bowl)*		1+			4
Sesame Oil *(Dynasty)*		1+			4
Sesame Oil *(KA-ME)*		1+			4
Sesame Oil *(Ty Ling)*		1+			4
Shells 'N Curry, Tofu Classics, Prepared, No Butter *(Fantastic Foods)*			2		
Soy Sauce *(Chun King)*			2+		
Soy Sauce *(Emperor's Kitchen)*			2+		
Soy Sauce *(Westbrae)*			2+		
Soy Sauce, Mild, 50% Less Sodium *(Westbrae)*			2+		
Soy Sauce, Organic *(Westbrae)*			2+		
Stir Fry Seasoning Mix *(S & B)*			2+		
Stir Fry Vegetables *(Dynasty)*	★				

1 = High Fat   2 = High Sodium   3 = High Refined Sugar   5 = Cholesterol
1+ = Very High Fat   2+ = Very High Sodium   4 = Highly Processed   ★= Better Choice

VARIETY *(Brand)*   RATING CODE

Sukiyaki, Seasoning Mix *(S & B)*	2+	
Sweet & Sour Sauce *(Kraft)*	2+	3
Sweet & Sour Sauce *(La Choy)*	2+	3
Sweet & Sour Sauce *(Sauceworks)*	2	3
Sweet & Sour Seasoning Mix *(S & B)*	2+	
Szechwan Seasoning Mix *(S & B)*	2+	
Tamari Sauce *(KA-ME)*	2+	
Tamari Sauce *(San-J)*	2+	
Tamari Sauce *(Westbrae)*	2+	
Tamari Sauce, Lite *(San-J)*	2+	
Tamari Soy Sauce *(Arrowhead Mills)*	2+	
Tamari, Wheat-Free *(Westbrae)*	2+	
Tempura Batter, Seasoning Mix *(S & B)*	2+	
Tofu *(Azumaya)*	1	
Tofu *(Frieda)*	1	
Tofu *(Hinoichi)*	1	
Tofu *(Mori-Nu)*	1	
Tofu *(MuTofu)*	1	
Tofu *(Soy Country)*	1	
Tofu Burger, Prepared *(Fantastic Foods)*	1	2
Tofu Scrambler, Prepared, No Butter *(Fantastic Foods)*	1	2
Tomato Beef Seasoning Mix *(S & B)*	2+	3
Vegetables, Chow Mein *(Chun King)*	★	
Vegetables, Mixed *(La Choy)*	2	
Vinegar, Natural Rice *(Nakano)*	★	
Vinegar, Red Rice *(China Bowl)*	★	
Vinegar, White Rice *(China Bowl)*	★	
Water Chestnuts *(China Bowl)*	★	
Water Chestnuts *(Chun King)*	★	
Water Chestnuts *(Green Giant)*	★	
Water Chestnuts *(La Choy)*	★	
Water Chestnuts *(Port Arthur)*	★	
Water Chestnuts *(Reese)*	★	

1 = High Fat	2 = High Sodium	3 = High Refined Sugar	5 = Cholesterol
1+ = Very High Fat	2+ = Very High Sodium	4 = Highly Processed	★= Better Choice

VARIETY *(Brand)*   RATING CODE

Water Chestnuts *(Roland)*	★
Water Chestnuts, Whole & Sliced *(Dynasty)*	★
Water Chestnuts, Whole & Sliced *(Fancifood)*	★

PANCAKE AND WAFFLE MIXES

I'm all for convenience when it comes to pancakes and waffles, so I keep these mixes on hand. Many brands, such as *Hungry Jack*, did not make *The Food Bible* largely because of aluminum. Personally, I use a whole grain mix such as *Arrowhead Mills* MultiGrain, then "doctor" it up by adding wheat germ and sunflower kernels or chopped pecans — and sometimes I will add raisins. This gives them a wonderful flavor plus it increases the nutrients and fiber.

VARIETY *(Brand)*   RATING CODE

PANCAKE AND WAFFLE MIXES		
Biscuit & Pancake Mix, Buttermilk *(Health Valley)*	2	
Pancake & Waffle Mix, Buckwheat *(Aunt Jemima)*	2+	
Pancake & Waffle Mix, Old-Fashioned *(Mrs. Butterworth's)*	2+	4
Pancake & Waffle Mix, Original *(Aunt Jemima)*	2+	4
Pancake & Waffle Mix, Whole Wheat *(Aunt Jemima)*	2+	
★ Pancake Mix, Blue Corn *(Arrowhead Mills)*		
Pancake Mix, Buckwheat *(Arrowhead Mills)*	2	
Pancake Mix, Buckwheat *(Hodgson Mill)*	2	
Pancake Mix, Griddle Lite *(Arrowhead Mills)*	2	
Pancake Mix, Multigrain *(Arrowhead Mills)*	2	
★ Pancake Mix, Oat Bran *(Arrowhead Mills)*		
Pancake Mix, Triticale *(Arrowhead Mills)*	2	
Pancake Mix, Whole Wheat Buttermilk *(Hodgson Mill)*	2	

---

1 = High Fat   2 = High Sodium   3 = High Refined Sugar   5 = Cholesterol
1+ = Very High Fat   2+ = Very High Sodium   4 = Highly Processed   ★= Better Choice

PASTA AND EGG NOODLES

I like pasta — no, I LOVE pasta. And I eat a lot of it. I'll top it with pasta sauces, use it in casseroles, in salads or anyplace else I can think of. I nearly always use whole grain pasta as it contains the whole grain which means more nutrients — including fiber. Pasta is an excellent source of complex carbohydrates, and as a group I rate it very high — particularly whole grain pasta.

VARIETY *(Brand)*   RATING CODE

PASTA AND EGG NOODLES		
EGG NOODLES: DRY		
Egg Noodles *(Ernte Dank)*	4	5
Egg Noodles *(Goodman's)*	4	5
Egg Noodles *(Greenfield's)*	4	5
Egg Noodles *(Hodgson Mill)*		5
Egg Noodles *(Inn Maid)*	4	5
Egg Noodles *(Light 'n Fluffy)*	4	5
Egg Noodles *(Mrs. Weiss)*	4	5
Egg Noodles *(No-Yolks)*	4	
EGG NOODLES: FROZEN		
Egg Noodles *(Reames)*	4	5
PASTA: DRY		
Pasta *(American Beauty)*	4	
Pasta *(Buitoni)*	4	
Pasta *(Creamette)*	4	
Pasta *(Da Vinci)*	4	
Pasta *(Dell' Alpe)*	4	
Pasta *(Edward & Sons)*	★	
Pasta *(Ferrara)*	4	
Pasta *(Fioota)*	4	
Pasta *(Globe "A1")*	4	
Pasta *(Golden Grain)*	4	
Pasta *(Health Valley)*	★	
Pasta *(Hodgson Mill)*	★	
Pasta *(Iberia)*	4	
Pasta *(Leonardo)*	4	
Pasta *(Martha Gooch)*	4	
Pasta *(Mrs. Leeper's)*	★	
Pasta *(Mueller's)*	4	
Pasta *(Perfection)*	4	
Pasta *(Ponte)*	4	
Pasta *(R-F)*	4	
Pasta *(Racconto)*	4	

VARIETY *(Brand)*   RATING CODE

Pasta *(Red Cross)*		4
Pasta *(Ronzoni)*		4
Pasta *(Rummo)*		4
Pasta *(San Giorgio)*		4
Pasta *(Silver Award)*		4
Pasta *(Skinner)*		4
Pasta *(Town House)*		4
Pasta, Artichoke *(DeBoles)*		4
Pasta, Corn *(DeBoles)*	★	
Pasta, Wheat *(DeBoles)*	★	

PASTA: REFRIGERATED
Pasta *(Contadina)*		4	5
Pasta *(Romance)*		4	5

PEANUT BUTTER AND OTHER BUTTERS

Peanut and other butters are like nuts and seeds — very nutritious but very high in fat. Some peanut butters, such as *Peter Pan* and *Skippy*, have added hydrogenated palm oil to make them spread more evenly and to keep the oil from separating. I could not put these varieties in *The Food Bible*. Peanut and other butters are very nutritious and tasty, but they need to be limited.

VARIETY *(Brand)*   RATING CODE

PEANUT BUTTER AND OTHER BUTTERS
PEANUT BUTTER
Peanut Butter *(East Wind)* — 1+
Peanut Butter *(Rainfall)* — 1+
Peanut Butter, Chunky & Creamy *(Country Pure)* — 1+

Peanut Butter, Chunky & Creamy *(Erewhon)* — 1+
Peanut Butter, Chunky & Creamy *(Smucker's)* — 1+
Peanut Butter, Chunky & Creamy, No Salt *(Health Valley)* — 1+

Peanut Butter, Chunky & Creamy, Unsalted *(Erewhon)* — 1+
Peanut Butter, Creamy & Crunchy *(Adams)* — 1+
Peanut Butter, Creamy & Crunchy *(Algood)* — 1+

Peanut Butter, Creamy, Natural *(Laura Scudder's)* — 1+
Peanut Butter, Crunchy & Creamy *(Arrowhead Mills)* — 1+
Peanut Butter, Crunchy & Creamy *(Gourmet Award)* — 1+

Peanut Butter, Crunchy & Creamy, No Salt *(R. W. Knudsen)* — 1+
Peanut Butter, Old-Fashioned *(Laura Scudder's)* — 1+ 2
Peanut Butter, Smooth & Crunchy *(Koeze's)* — 1+

Peanut Butter, Unsalted *(Adams)* — 1+

OTHER BUTTERS
Almond Butter *(Erewhon)* — 1+
Almond Butter *(Maranatha)* — 1+

Almond Butter, Creamy & Crunchy *(California)* — 1+
Almond Butter, Natural Raw *(Hain)* — 1+
Almond Butter, Toasted & Blanched *(Hain)* — 1+

Cashew Butter *(Erewhon)* — 1+
Cashew Butter, Raw *(Hain)* — 1+
Cashew Butter, Toasted *(Hain)* — 1+

Sesame Butter *(Erewhon)* — 1+
Sesame Tahini *(Arrowhead Mills)* — 1+
Sesame Tahini *(Erewhon)* — 1+

Sunflower Butter *(Erewhon)* — 1+
Tahini Butter *(Fantis)* — 1+

1 = High Fat   2 = High Sodium   3 = High Refined Sugar   5 = Cholesterol
1+ = Very High Fat   2+ = Very High Sodium   4 = Highly Processed   ★= Better Choice

RICE

This is an extremely healthful food in its original form, which is brown rice. White rice is a highly processed food, which means it has very little fiber and many valuable vitamins and minerals are lost. Nearly all brands of boxed rice dinners contain additives and preservatives. For example: *Rice-A-Roni* Savory Classics, Broccoli au Gratin contains MSG, artificial flavor, BHA, sodium sulfite, sodium bisulfite and propyl gallate.

I rate white rice a little over white bread and white flour. Our best choice by far is brown rice. On the other hand, I understand the problem — brown rice does take longer to prepare, and it's almost impossible to get it in a restaurant. We're seeing quite a few brands of quick brown rice these days. It is good — both good tasting as well as nutritious. But it still is not as nutritious as regular brown rice — nor as tasty, in my opinion. But I do keep it on hand for those days when there just isn't time to cook the regular brown rice. It truly is quick and easy as well as nutritious.

VARIETY *(Brand)*   RATING CODE

RICE
BOXED

Variety (Brand)	Rating Code
Aromatic Long Grain *(Uncle Ben's)*	4
Aromatic Long Grain, Boil-In-Bag *(Uncle Ben's)*	4
Basmati *(Fantastic Foods)*	4
Beef Flavored Rice *(Near East)*	2 4
Boil-In-Bag *(Uncle Ben's)*	4
Brown, Boil-In-Bag *(Success)*	★
Brown, Fast Cooking *(Uncle Ben's)*	★
Brown, Instant *(Minute)*	★
Brown, Quick Cooking *(Arrowhead Mills)*	★
Brown, 10-Minute *(Gourmet Award)*	★
Instant *(Uncle Ben's)*	4
Long Grain & Wild, Garden Vegetable Blend *(Uncle Ben's)*	2+ 4
Long Grain, Microwave *(Uncle Ben's)*	4
Minute Rice *(Minute)*	4

BROWN

Variety (Brand)	Rating Code
Brown Rice *(Arrowhead Mills)*	★
Brown Rice *(Comet)*	★
Brown Rice *(Fantastic Foods)*	★
Brown Rice *(Hinode)*	★
Brown Rice *(Homai)*	★
Brown Rice *(Konriko)*	★
Brown Rice *(Lundberg)*	★
Brown Rice *(Mahatma)*	★
Brown Rice *(Riceland)*	★
Brown Rice *(S & W)*	★
Brown Rice *(Stone-Buhr)*	★
Brown Rice *(Termati)*	★
Brown Rice *(Town House)*	★
Brown Rice *(Uncle Ben's)*	★

WHITE

Variety (Brand)	Rating Code
White Rice *(Adolphus)*	4
White Rice *(Big Chief)*	4
White Rice *(Canilla)*	4

1 = High Fat
1+ = Very High Fat
2 = High Sodium
2+ = Very High Sodium
3 = High Refined Sugar
4 = Highly Processed
5 = Cholesterol
★ = Better Choice

VARIETY *(Brand)*   RATING CODE

White Rice *(Comet)*	4
White Rice *(Dynasty)*	4
White Rice *(Evans)*	4
White Rice *(Fiesta)*	4
White Rice *(Goya)*	4
White Rice *(Hinode)*	4
White Rice *(Iberia)*	4
White Rice *(Mahatma)*	4
White Rice *(Mandarin)*	4
White Rice *(Martha White)*	4
White Rice *(Rainbow)*	4
White Rice *(Riceland)*	4
White Rice *(Success)*	4
White Rice *(Tender Cook)*	4
White Rice *(Uncle Ben's)*	4
White Rice *(Vigo)*	4
White Rice *(Vitarroz)*	4
White Rice *(Water Maid)*	4
WILD	
Wild Rice *(Fantastic Foods)*	★
Wild Rice *(Gourmet Award)*	★
Wild Rice *(Gourmet House)*	★
Wild Rice *(Gourmet Valley)*	★
Wild Rice *(Reese)*	★

1 = High Fat	2 = High Sodium	3 = High Refined Sugar	5 = Cholesterol
1+ = Very High Fat	2+ = Very High Sodium	4 = Highly Processed	★= Better Choice

SALAD DRESSINGS

Most all salad dressings won't add much to our health status, but they sure do make our taste buds dance. Fat, salt, sugar — salad dressings can have them all. Additives and preservatives also run rampant. For example: *Kraft* Ranch-Free (Fat Free and Cholesterol Free) contains MSG, potassium sorbate, EDTA, propylene glycol alginate and artificial color. *Seven Seas* Creamy Italian contains polysorbate 60, artificial color, EDTA and yellow #5. I've eliminated dressings such as these from *The Food Bible*, but most that are included are not very healthful.

I really don't feel that salad dressings were designed to be food anyway. They're used to enhance the flavor of food — and have they ever been a good seller! If we could get back to the herbal concept of salad seasoning, we would be better off. *Pritikin* markets French and Italian products of this nature that I like, and there are other good ones. Since I know that most of us are going to use salad dressings, don't miss the trick I use to get the taste without the volume.

Have your dressing in a *small* container at the side of your salad plate. Spear a bite of salad, then *barely* touch the tip of your salad to the dressing. By doing this, the first flavor your taste buds sense is the dressing, and this tiny amount is all that it will take to satisfy you.

VARIETY *(Brand)*   RATING CODE

	Rating Code
SALAD DRESSINGS	
Bleu Cheese *(Litehouse)*	1+ 2+
Blue Cheese *(Marie's)*	1+ 2+
Blue Cheese Mix, Prepared *(Mayacamas)*	1+
Buttermilk, Old-Fashioned *(Hain)*	1+ 2
Buttermilk, Old-Fashioned *(Hollywood)*	1+ 2
Caesar, Creamy *(Hain)*	1+ 2+
Caesar, Creamy, Low Salt *(Hain)*	1+
Caesar, Original *(Cardini's)*	1+ 2+
Champagne Mustard *(Cuisine Pérel)*	1+ 2
Cheese & Garlic *(Bernstein's)*	1+ 2
Country Style *(Litehouse)*	1+ 2+
Cucumber Dill *(Hain)*	1+ 2
French *(Mullen's)*	1+ 2
French *(Pritikin)*	★
French Country Herb *(Litehouse)*	1+ 2+
French, California *(Marzetti)*	1+ 2
French, Creamy *(Hain)*	1+
Garden Herb, Vegi-Dressing *(Nasoya)*	1+
Garlic & Cheese *(Anne's Vermont)*	1+ 2
Garlic & Sour Cream *(Hain)*	1+ 2
Garlic Dill *(Cuisine Pérel)*	1+ 2
Garlic, Lemon & Dill Mix, Prepared *(Mayacamas)*	1+ 2
Herb Basket, Reduced Calorie *(Mrs. Pickford's)*	2+
Herb French, The Source *(Cardini's)*	1+ 2
Herb, Savory, No Salt Added *(Hain)*	1+
Honey & Sesame *(Hain)*	1+ 2+
Italian *(Bernstein's)*	1+ 2
Italian *(Cardini's)*	1+ 2+
Italian *(Pritikin)*	★
Italian *(Richard Simmons)*	1+ 2+
Italian *(Sutter Home)*	1+ 2
Italian with Cheese *(Bernstein's)*	1+ 2
Italian, Creamy *(Hain)*	1+

1 = High Fat	2 = High Sodium	3 = High Refined Sugar	5 = Cholesterol
1+ = Very High Fat	2+ = Very High Sodium	4 = Highly Processed	★= Better Choice

VARIETY *(Brand)*   RATING CODE

VARIETY (Brand)	RATING CODE
Italian, Creamy *(Marie's)*	1+ 2+
Italian, Creamy, No Salt Added *(Hain)*	1+
Italian, Mix *(Lawry's)*	2+ 3
Italian, No Oil Mix *(Good Seasons)*	2+ 3
Italian, No Salt *(Cardini's)*	1+
Italian, Traditional *(Hain)*	1+ 2+
Italian, Traditional, No Salt Added *(Hain)*	1+
Italian, Vegi-Dressing *(Nasoya)*	1+
Lemon Chardonnay *(Cuisine Pérel)*	1+ 2
Lemon Herb *(Cardini's)*	1+ 2+
Lemon Herb, No Salt *(Cardini's)*	1+
Lime Dill *(Cardini's)*	1+ 2
Mayonnaise, Cold-Pressed *(Hain)*	1+
Mayonnaise, Eggless, No Salt Added *(Hain)*	1+
Mayonnaise, Light, Low Sodium *(Hain)*	1+ 2
Mayonnaise, No Salt *(Hain)*	1+
Mayonnaise, Real, No Salt Added *(Hain)*	1+
Mayonnaise, Safflower *(Hain)*	1+
Miracle Whip *(Kraft)*	1+
Miracle Whip Light *(Kraft)*	1+ 2
Miracle Whip Light, Cholesterol Free *(Kraft)*	1+ 2
Miracle Whip, Cholesterol Free *(Kraft)*	1+ 2
No Oil 1000 Island Mix, Prepared *(Hain)*	2+
No Oil Bleu Cheese Mix, Prepared *(Hain)*	2+
No Oil Buttermilk Mix, Prepared *(Hain)*	2+
No Oil Caesar Mix, Prepared *(Hain)*	2+
No Oil French Mix, Prepared *(Hain)*	2+
No Oil Garlic & Cheese Mix, Prepared *(Hain)*	2+
No Oil Herb Mix, Prepared *(Hain)*	2+
No Oil Italian Mix, Prepared *(Hain)*	2+
Oil & Vinegar *(Newman's Own)*	1+ 2+
Olive Oil Dressing, Creamy *(Bertolli)*	1+ 2+
Olive Oil Dressing, Original *(Bertolli)*	1+ 2

1 = High Fat   2 = High Sodium   3 = High Refined Sugar   5 = Cholesterol
1+ = Very High Fat   2+ = Very High Sodium   4 = Highly Processed   ★= Better Choice

VARIETY *(Brand)*   **RATING CODE**

Olive Oil Dressing, Zesty *(Bertolli)*	1+ 2+
Pesto Pasta *(Cardini's)*	1+ 2+
Poppy Seed *(Litehouse)*	1+ 2+ 3
Poppyseed Rancher's *(Hain)*	1+ 2 3
Ranch *(Litehouse)*	1+ 2+
Roma Cheese *(Richard Simmons)*	1+ 2+
Russian *(Pritikin)*	★
Sandwich & Salad Sauce *(Durkee)*	1+ 2+
Sesame Garlic, Vegi-Dressing *(Nasoya)*	1+
Sicilian Style Dressing & Marinade *(Arbisi's)*	1+ 2+
Slaw Dressing, Light *(Marzetti's)*	1+ 2+ 3
Slaw Dressing, Original *(Marzetti's)*	1+ 2+ 3
Sour Cream & Dill *(Marie's)*	1+ 2+
Sweet & Sour *(Maple Grove Farms)*	1+ 2 3
Sweet & Sour *(Mrs. Pickford's)*	2+ 3
1000 Island *(Hain)*	1+ 2
Thousand Island *(Hollywood)*	1+ 2
Thousand Island *(Litehouse)*	1+ 2 3
Tomato *(Pritikin)*	★
Vinaigrette *(Pritikin)*	★
Vinaigrette, Dijon *(Hain)*	1+ 2+
Vinaigrette, Honey Herb Mix, Prepared *(Mayacamas)*	1+ 3
Vinaigrette, Italian Cheese *(Hain)*	1+ 2
Vinaigrette, Italian Mix, Prepared *(Mayacamas)*	1+
Vinaigrette, Reduced Calorie *(Mrs. Pickford's)*	2+
Vinaigrette, Swiss Cheese *(Hain)*	1+ 2
Zesty Tomato, Reduced Calorie *(Mrs. Pickford's)*	2+ 3

1 = High Fat	2 = High Sodium	3 = High Refined Sugar	5 = Cholesterol
1+ = Very High Fat	2+ = Very High Sodium	4 = Highly Processed	★= Better Choice

SAUCES

Most all sauces are high in sodium. As an example, *Hunt's* Tomato Sauce has 670 mg. of sodium for 1/2 cup. There are some no-salt varieties in *The Food Bible*, and these are a better choice. As for spaghetti sauce, it is usually high in sodium. Most varieties are free of additives and preservatives, but some will contain cottonseed oil — such as *Prego*. Some other sauces contain additives which I feel are harmful, such as sodium benzoate and potassium sorbate found in *Heinz 57 Sauce*.

There are many sauces that made *The Food Bible*. Just be aware of the high sodium content in most of them.

VARIETY *(Brand)*   RATING CODE

SAUCES
BOTTLED AND CANNED

Variety (Brand)	Rating Code
Cajun Cooking Sauce *(S & W)*	2+
Chili Sauce *(Bennett's)*	2+ 3
Chili Sauce *(Heinz)*	2+ 3
Chocolate Sauce, No Sugar *(Chocolate Mountain)*	1
Clam Sauce, Red *(Da Vinci)*	1 2+
Clam Sauce, White *(Buitoni)*	1+ 2+
Cranberry Sauce, Jellied *(R. W. Knudsen)*	★
Cranberry Sauce, Natural *(R. W. Knudsen)*	★
Creole Mustard Sauce *(New Orleans Jubilee)*	2+
Extra Thick & Chunky Sauce, Manwich *(Hunt's)*	2+ 3
Hollandaise Sauce, Cajun *(New Orleans Jubilee)*	2+
Hot Fudge Topping *(R & R Homestead)*	1 3
Marinara Sauce *(Progresso)*	1 2+
Marinara Spaghetti Sauce *(Buitoni)*	2+
Meat Loaf Sauce *(Compliment)*	2+
Mint Sauce *(Crosse & Blackwell)*	3
Not-So-Sloppy Joe Sauce *(Hormel)*	2+ 3
Pasta Sauce *(Ci' Bella)*	2
Pasta Sauce *(Sutter Home)*	1 2+
Pasta Sauce *(Tree of Life)*	1 2+
Pasta Sauce, Beef & Pork *(Classico)*	1+ 2+
Pasta Sauce, Beef & Vegetable *(Classico)*	1+ 2+
Pasta Sauce, Italian, Hot & Spicy *(Ragu)*	1 2+ 3
Pasta Sauce, Italian, Mushrooms *(Ragu)*	1 2+ 3
Pasta Sauce, Italian, Parmesan *(Ragu)*	1 2+ 3
Pasta Sauce, Italian, Tomato, Herb *(Ragu)*	1 2+ 3
Pasta Sauce, Ripe Olive & Mushroom *(Classico)*	1 2+
Pasta Sauce, Shrimp & Crab *(Classico)*	1 2+ 5
Pasta Sauce, Spicy Red Pepper *(Classico)*	1 2+
Pasta Sauce, Tomato & Basil *(Classico)*	1+ 2+
Pizza Quick Sauce, Traditional *(Ragu)*	1 2+
Pizza Sauce *(Don Pepino)*	1 2+
Pizza Sauce *(Enrico's)*	1 2+

1 = High Fat   2 = High Sodium   3 = High Refined Sugar   5 = Cholesterol
1+ = Very High Fat   2+ = Very High Sodium   4 = Highly Processed   ★= Better Choice

VARIETY *(Brand)*   RATING CODE

VARIETY (Brand)	★	1	2+	3
Pizza Sauce *(Progresso)*		1	2+	
Pizza Sauce *(Ragu)*		1	2+	
Pizza Sauce with Cheese *(Chef Boyardee)*		1+	2+	
Raisin Sauce *(Chelten House)*				3
Seafood Cocktail Sauce *(Crosse & Blackwell)*			2+	3
Seafood Cocktail Sauce *(Del Monte)*			2+	3
Seafood Cocktail Sauce *(Heinz)*			2+	3
Seafood Cocktail Sauce *(Reese)*			2+	3
Seafood Cocktail Sauce *(S & W)*			2+	3
Shrimp Sauce *(Crosse & Blackwell)*			2+	3
Sloppy Joe *(Libby's)*			2+	3
Sloppy Joe Sandwich Sauce *(Aunt Nellie's)*			2+	
Sloppy Joe Sauce, Manwich *(Hunt's)*			2+	3
Spaghetti Sauce *(Enrico's)*			2+	
Spaghetti Sauce *(Johnson's)*			2+	
Spaghetti Sauce *(Newman's Own)*		1	2+	
Spaghetti Sauce *(Pritikin)*	★			
Spaghetti Sauce with Meat *(Buitoni)*		1	2+	
Spaghetti Sauce with Meat *(Chef Boyardee)*		1	2+	
Spaghetti Sauce with Meat *(Hunt's)*		1	2+	3
Spaghetti Sauce with Meat *(Progresso)*		1	2+	
Spaghetti Sauce with Meat *(Rainbow)*		1	2+	
Spaghetti Sauce with Meat *(Weight Watchers)*			2+	
Spaghetti Sauce with Mushrooms *(Mama Cocco's)*	★			
Spaghetti Sauce with Mushrooms *(Pritikin)*	★			
Spaghetti Sauce with Mushrooms *(Weight Watchers)*			2+	
Spaghetti Sauce, Extra Virgin *(Venecia)*			2+	3
Spaghetti Sauce, Gardenstyle with Peppers & Mushrooms *(Ragu)*			2+	
Spaghetti Sauce, Gardenstyle, Extra Tomato, Garlic & Onion *(Ragu)*			2+	
Spaghetti Sauce, Gardenstyle, Mushroom & Onions *(Ragu)*			2+	
Spaghetti Sauce, Homestyle *(Hunt's)*			2+	3
Spaghetti Sauce, Homestyle Mushroom *(Ragu)*			2+	
Spaghetti Sauce, Homestyle Natural *(Ragu)*			2+	

1 = High Fat	2 = High Sodium	3 = High Refined Sugar	5 = Cholesterol
1+ = Very High Fat	2+ = Very High Sodium	4 = Highly Processed	★ = Better Choice

VARIETY *(Brand)*   RATING CODE

Spaghetti Sauce, Homestyle with Meat *(Ragu)*		2+	
Spaghetti Sauce, Homestyle, No Sugar *(Hunt's)*		2+	
Spaghetti Sauce, Low Sodium *(Eden)*	1		
Spaghetti Sauce, Marinara, No Salt *(Mama Cocco's)*	1		
Spaghetti Sauce, Meat *(Ragu)*		2+	
Spaghetti Sauce, Mushroom *(Buitoni)*	1	2+	
Spaghetti Sauce, Mushroom *(Hunt's)*	1	2+	3
Spaghetti Sauce, Mushroom *(Progresso)*	1	2+	
Spaghetti Sauce, Mushroom *(Rainbow)*		2+	
Spaghetti Sauce, Natural *(Progresso)*	1	2+	
Spaghetti Sauce, Natural *(Ragu)*	1	2+	
Spaghetti Sauce, Plain *(Rainbow)*	1	2+	
Spaghetti Sauce, Sockarooni *(Newman's Own)*		2+	
Spaghetti Sauce, Thick & Hearty Meat *(Ragu)*		2+	
Spaghetti Sauce, Thick & Hearty Natural *(Ragu)*	1	2+	
Spaghetti Sauce, Thick & Hearty with Mushrooms *(Ragu)*	1	2+	
Spaghetti Sauce, Traditional *(Hunt's)*	1	2+	3
Steak & Chop Sauce *(London Pub)*		2+	
Steak Sauce *(A.1.)*		2+	
Steak Sauce *(Mrs. Dash)*	★		
Steak Sauce *(Prime Choice)*		2+	
Steak Sauce, H. P. *(Lea & Perrins)*		2+	
Sweet 'n Sour Sauce *(Sauceworks)*		2	3
Tomato Paste *(Contadina)*	★		
Tomato Paste *(Del Monte)*	★		
Tomato Paste *(Hunt's)*		2	
Tomato Paste *(Town House)*	★		
Tomato Paste with Garlic *(Hunt's)*		2+	
Tomato Paste, Italian Style *(Hunt's)*		2+	
Tomato Puree, No Salt *(Progresso)*	★		
Tomato Sauce *(Contadina)*		2+	
Tomato Sauce *(Del Monte)*		2+	
Tomato Sauce *(El Pato)*		2+	

1 = High Fat	2 = High Sodium	3 = High Refined Sugar	5 = Cholesterol
1+ = Very High Fat	2+ = Very High Sodium	4 = Highly Processed	★= Better Choice

VARIETY *(Brand)*   RATING CODE

Tomato Sauce *(Health Valley)*		2+		
Tomato Sauce *(Hunt's)*		2+		
Tomato Sauce *(Iberia)*		2+		
Tomato Sauce *(Progresso)*		2+		
Tomato Sauce *(Rainbow)*		2+		
Tomato Sauce *(Town House)*		2+		
Tomato Sauce, Garlic *(Hunt's)*		2+		
Tomato Sauce, Italian Style *(Contadina)*		2+		
Tomato Sauce, Meat Loaf Fixin's *(Hunt's)*		2+		
Tomato Sauce, No Salt *(Del Monte)*	★			
Tomato Sauce, No Salt *(Health Valley)*	★			
Tomato Sauce, Special *(Hunt's)*		2+		
Tomato Sauce, Thick & Zesty *(Contadina)*		2+		
White Sauce *(Aunt Penny's)*	1+	2+		
FROZEN				
Alfredo Sauce *(Putney Pasta)*	1+	2		5
Pesto Sauce *(Putney Pasta)*	1+	2		5
Shrimp Sauce *(Sau Sea)*		2+	3	
Walnut Sauce *(Putney Pasta)*	1+			
MIXES				
Alfredo Sauce Mix, Prepared *(Mayacamas)*	1+			5
Brown Gravy Mix *(Knorr)*		2+		
Clam, Creamy Pasta Sauce Mix, Prepared *(Mayacamas)*	1+			5
Hollandaise Sauce Mix, Prepared *(Knorr)*		2+		
Honey Mustard Sauce Mix, Prepared *(Mayacamas)*	1+			
Hunter Sauce Mix *(Knorr)*		2+		
Lyonnaise Sauce Mix, Prepared *(Knorr)*	1	2+		
Mushroom Sauce Mix, Prepared *(Knorr)*	1	2+		
Newburg Sauce Mix, Prepared *(Knorr)*	1	2+		
Pesto Sauce Mix, Prepared *(Mayacamas)*	1+			5
Spaghetti Sauce, Napoli, Prepared *(Knorr)*	1+	2+		

1 = High Fat	2 = High Sodium	3 = High Refined Sugar	5 = Cholesterol
1+ = Very High Fat	2+ = Very High Sodium	4 = Highly Processed	★= Better Choice

VARIETY *(Brand)*   RATING CODE

REFRIGERATED	
Alfredo Sauce *(Contadina)*	1+ 5
Creamy Dijon *(Contadina)*	1+ 2+ 5
Forestiera Sauce *(Contadina)*	2+
Four Cheese Sauce *(Contadina)*	1+ 5
Marinara Sauce *(Contadina)*	1+ 2+
Marinara Sauce *(Romance)*	1+ 2+
Plum Sauce *(Contadina)*	1+ 2+
Primavera Sauce *(Contadina)*	1+ 2+
Tomato Alfresco *(Contadina)*	1+ 2+

SEASONING MIXES

Oh, boy! The majority of these are crammed with things that cause our body to say "ouch." Many contain additives and preservatives. Let's look at a few products and at the additives and preservatives they contain:

Lawry's Beef Marinade	MSG
French's Spaghetti Sauce Mix	sodium sulfite
Durkee Chicken Gravy Mix	MSG, disodium inosinate, disodium guanylate and artificial color

I will use seasoning mixes at times to give that special flavor to certain dishes. But since most seasoning mixes are so high in sodium, I take care not to add salt to the rest of the meal.

VARIETY *(Brand)*   RATING CODE

SEASONING MIXES
Alfredo Pasta Sauce *(Old Monk)*		2+
Au Jus Gravy Mix, Prepared *(Knorr)*	1	2+
Bean Seasoning Mix *(Wick Fowler's)*	★	

Brown Gravy Mix *(Lawry's)*	2+
Brown Gravy Mix *(Williams)*	2+
Brown Gravy Mix, Prepared *(Knorr)*	2+

Chili Mix *(Carroll Shelby's)*		2+
Chili Mix *(Durkee)*		2+
Chili Mix *(La Preferida)*	★	

Chili Mix *(Lawry's)*	2+
Chili Mix *(Mickey Gilley's)*	2+
Chili Mix *(Tio Sancho)*	2+

Chili Mix *(Williams)*	★	
Chili Mix with Onion *(Williams)*	★	
Chili Mix, Family Style, Mild *(Wick Fowler's)*		2+

Chili Mix, Mild & Hot *(McCormick)*		2+
Chili Mix, Tex-Mex *(Williams)*	★	
Chili Mix, Texas Red *(Durkee)*		2+

Chili Mix, Turkey *(Williams)*	★	
Chili Mix, Vegetarian *(Fantastic Foods)*		2
Chili Mixin's, Six Gun *(OL' I lired I land's)*		2

Chili, 2-Alarm *(Wick Fowler's)*	2+
Enchilada Sauce Mix *(McCormick)*	2+
Fajita Seasoning Mix *(Casa Fiesta)*	2+

Sloppy Joe Manwich Mix *(Hunt's)*	2+
Sloppy Joe Seasoning Mix *(Hunt's)*	2+
Spaghetti Sauce Mix *(Williams)*	2+ 3

Taco Seasoning Mix *(el Rio)*	2+
Taco Seasoning Mix *(French's)*	2+
Taco Seasoning Mix *(Lawry's)*	2+

Taco Seasoning Mix *(Tio Sancho)*	2+
Taco Seasoning Mix *(Wick Fowler's)*	2+
Taco Seasoning Mix *(Williams)*	2+

1 = High Fat   2 = High Sodium   3 = High Refined Sugar   5 = Cholesterol
1+ = Very High Fat   2+ = Very High Sodium   4 = Highly Processed   ★= Better Choice

VARIETY *(Brand)*   RATING CODE

Taco Seasoning Mix, Tex-Mex *(Williams)*	2+

SNACKS

Every "quick stop" in America is loaded with all kinds of snacks that sell for elevated prices and fuel a very profitable industry.

One of the definitions for a "junk bond" is high risk. Well, I think that is also the definition for "junk food." Many of us find ourselves developing habits such as eating junk food, and then suddenly we wake up and ask, "How did I get started doing this?" If you haven't been there, you're lucky.

I do see some good things happening in the snack industry. Companies such as *Health Valley*, *Barbara's*, *Natures Warehouse*, and others are certainly giving us a choice. These type products are quite superior to most of what is on the market. These products are much lower in fat and sodium, and many do not use refined sugars, and most are not highly processed. They are still snacks and should not be confused with meals, but they can be a tremendous choice for snacks. If you're one of many in our society who is hooked on chips and Twinkies, you can now upgrade the quality of your snacks. For example: *Health Valley* Blueberry Muffins certainly are a lot better than a donut from the donut shop on the way to work in the mornings.

VARIETY *(Brand)*   RATING CODE

SNACKS

Variety (Brand)	★	1	2	3	4	5
Apple Bakes *(Health Valley)*				3		
Blue Corn Curls, Salted *(Arrowhead Mills)*			2			
Blue Corn Curls, Unsalted *(Arrowhead Mills)*	★					
Carrot Chips *(Hain)*		1+				
Carrot Chips, No Salt Added *(Hain)*		1				
Carrot Lites *(Health Valley)*	★					
Cheddar Lites *(Health Valley)*		1				
Cheddar Lites, Green Onions *(Health Valley)*	★					
Cheddar Lites, No Salt *(Health Valley)*		1				
Cheese Puffs, Original *(Barbara's)*	★					
Corn Cakes, No Sodium *(Quaker)*					4	
Corn Chips *(Arrowhead Mills)*			2			
Corn Chips *(Fritos)*		1+	2			
Corn Chips with Cheese *(Arrowhead Mills)*			2			
Corn Chips, Cheddar Cheese *(Health Valley)*		1+				
Corn Chips, Crisp 'n Thin *(Frito Lay)*		1+	2			
Corn Chips, No Salt *(Health Valley)*		1+				
Corn Crisps, Corn Flavor *(Pringles)*		1	2			
Date Bakes *(Health Valley)*				3		
Fromage Sticks, Cheddar *(Select Harvest)*			2			
Fromage Sticks, Pesto *(Select Harvest)*			2			
Fruit & Fitness Bars *(Health Valley)*				3		
Fruit Bars, Apple *(Nature's Choice)*	★					
Fruit Bars, Apple *(Sunfield)*				3		
Fruit Bars, Apricot *(Nature's Choice)*	★					
Fruit Bars, Apricot *(Sunfield)*				3		
Fruit Bars, Cherry *(Nature's Choice)*	★					
Fruit Bars, Cherry *(Sunfield)*				3		
Fruit Bars, Grape *(Nature's Choice)*	★					
Fruit Bars, Grape *(Sunfield)*				3		
Fruit Bars, Raspberry *(Nature's Choice)*	★					
Fruit Bars, Raspberry *(Sunfield)*				3		
Fruit Bars, Strawberry *(Sunfield)*				3		

1 = High Fat   2 = High Sodium   3 = High Refined Sugar   5 = Cholesterol
1+ = Very High Fat   2+ = Very High Sodium   4 = Highly Processed   ★= Better Choice

VARIETY (Brand) — RATING CODE

VARIETY (Brand)	★	1 / 1+	2	3	4
Graham Bites, Brown Sugar 'n Spice (Nabisco)				3	4
Graham Bites, Honey 'n Oat Bran (Nabisco)				3	4
Granola Bars Light, Apricot (Barbara's)	★				
Granola Bars Light, Blueberry (Barbara's)	★				
Granola Bars Light, Raspberry (Barbara's)	★				
Granola Bars with Almonds (Little Debbie)		1		3	
Granola Bars with Raisins (Little Debbie)		1		3	
Granola Bars, Carob Chip (Nature's Choice)				3	
Granola Bars, Chocolate Chip (Little Debbie)		1		3	
Granola Bars, Cinnamon & Oats (Barbara's)		1			
Granola Bars, Cinnamon & Raisin (Nature's Choice)				3	
Granola Bars, Oats 'n Honey (Little Debbie)		1		3	
Granola Bars, Oats 'n Honey (Nature's Choice)				3	
Granola Bars, Peanut Butter (Barbara's)		1			
Granola Bars, Peanut Butter (Nature's Choice)		1		3	
Granola Bars, Rice Bran (Nature Valley)		1		3	4
Halvah, Carob Sesame (Fantastic Foods)		1		3	
Halvah, Cashew Currant (Fantastic Foods)		1		3	
Halvah, Sesame Honey (Fantastic Foods)		1		3	
Ideal Bars, Date-N-Orange (Thompson Foods)				3	
Ideal Bars, Green Apple (Thompson Foods)				3	
Ideal Bars, Peaches & Spice (Thompson Foods)				3	
Mexican Crisps (Old El Paso)		1+		3	4
Muffins, Apple Oatmeal Spice (Food for Life)		1		3	
Muffins, Banana (Food for Life)		1		3	
Muffins, Banana Nut (Pepperidge Farm)		1		3	4
Muffins, Bran with Raisins (Pepperidge Farm)		1	2	3	4
Muffins, Fancy Fruit, Almond & Date (Health Valley)	★				
Muffins, Fancy Fruit, Blueberry (Health Valley)	★				
Muffins, Fancy Fruit, Raisin (Health Valley)	★				
Muffins, Oat Bran & Apples (Pepperidge Farm)		1		3	4
Muffins, Raisin Bran (Food for Life)		1		3	
Muffins, Rice Bran, Raisin (Health Valley)	★				

1 = High Fat   2 = High Sodium   3 = High Refined Sugar   5 = Cholesterol
1+ = Very High Fat   2+ = Very High Sodium   4 = Highly Processed   ★= Better Choice

VARIETY (Brand) — RATING CODE

VARIETY (Brand)	★	1	2	3	4
Multi-Grain Cakes *(Quaker)*	★				
Munchies, Chocolate Fudge *(Skinny Haven)*				3	
Munchies, Nacho Cheese *(Skinny Haven)*		1	2		
Munchies, Onion *(Skinny Haven)*		1	2		
Nachips *(Old El Paso)*		1			
Nacho Chips *(Authentic)*		1			
Nacho Chips, No Salt *(La Preferida)*		1			
Nachos, No Salt *(Authentic)*		1+			
Oat Bran Apricot Bakes *(Health Valley)*				3	
Oat Bran Bars, Apple Cinnamon *(Nature's Choice)*	★				
Oat Bran Bars, Mixed Fruit *(Nature's Choice)*	★				
Oat Bran Bars, Triple Bran with Apricot *(Nature's Choice)*	★				
Oat Bran Fig & Nut Bakes *(Health Valley)*				3	
Oat Bran Fruit Bars, Almond & Date *(Health Valley)*	★				
Oat Bran Fruit Bars, Fruit & Nut *(Health Valley)*	★				
Oat Bran Fruit Bars, Raisin & Cinnamon *(Health Valley)*	★				
Oat Bran Jumbo Fruit Bars *(Health Valley)*	★				
Pastry Popper, Apple *(Natures Warehouse)*	★				
Pastry Popper, Strawberry *(Natures Warehouse)*	★				
Peanut Butter Crunch *(Barbara's)*		1		3	
Popcorn Cakes *(Quaker)*			2		4
Popcorn Cakes, Butter Flavor *(Quaker)*			2		4
Popcorn Cakes, Sesame *(Chico San)*	★				
Popcorn, Micro *(Pops-Rite)*		1	2		
Popcorn, Micro *(Weight Watchers)*	★				
Popcorn, Microwave, Light Natural *(Orville Redenbacher)*			2+		
Popcorn, Microwave, Natural *(Orville Redenbacher)*		1+	2+		
Popcorn, Microwave, Natural Butter Flavor *(Newman's Own)*		1			
Popcorn, Microwave, Natural Flavor *(Newman's Own)*		1			
Popcorn, Microwave, Natural, Salt Free *(Orville Redenbacher)*		1+			
Popcorn, Natural *(raw kernels)*	★				
Popcorn, Popped Cheddar Cheese *(Smartfood)*		1+	2		
Popcorn, White, Popped *(Vic's)*		1+	2		

1 = High Fat   2 = High Sodium   3 = High Refined Sugar   5 = Cholesterol
1+ = Very High Fat   2+ = Very High Sodium   4 = Highly Processed   ★ = Better Choice

VARIETY (Brand) — RATING CODE

VARIETY (Brand)	★				
Potato Chips, Country (Health Valley)		1+			
Potato Chips, Country, No Salt (Health Valley)		1+			
Potato Chips, Country Ripple (Health Valley)		1+			
Potato Chips, Country Ripple, No Salt (Health Valley)		1+			
Potato Chips, Dip (Health Valley)		1+			
Potato Chips, Dip, No Salt (Health Valley)		1+			
Potato Chips, Groovy ("Mike-sell's")		1+			
Potato Chips, Natural (Health Valley)		1+			
Potato Chips, Natural, No Salt (Health Valley)		1+			
Potato Chips, Old-Fashioned ("Mike-sell's")		1+			
Potato Chips, Original (Krunchers)		1+			
Potato Chips, Plain Kettle Style (Vegas Chips)		1+	2		
Potato Chips, Regular ("Mike-sell's")		1+			
Pretzels (Dutch Country)			2+		4
Pretzels, Butter (Seyfert's)			2+		4
Pretzels, Mini-Twist (Laura Scudder's)			2+		4
Pretzels, Oat Bran Nuggets (Pennysticks)			2+		4
Pretzels, Sourdough (Wege)			2+		4
Pretzels, Sourdough, Unsalted (Snyder's)					4
Pretzels, Sticks (Laura Scudder's)			2+		4
Pretzels, Twists (Laura Scudder's)			2+		4
Pretzels, Unsalted (Wege)					4
Pretzels, Whole Wheat (Barbara's)			2		
Pretzels, Whole Wheat, Unsalted (Wege)	★				
Raisin Bakes (Health Valley)				3	
Rice Bran Fruit Bars, Almond & Date (Health Valley)	★				
Rice Cakes (Quaker)	★				
Rice Cakes, Brown Rice, Low Sodium (Lundberg)			2		
Rice Cakes, Brown Rice, Sodium Free (Lundberg)	★				
Rice Cakes, Double Sesame (Westbrae Natural)			2		
Rice Cakes, 5-Grain (Hain)	★				
Rice Cakes, Mini Apple Cinnamon (Hain)	★				
Rice Cakes, Mini Cheese (Hain)	★				

1 = High Fat   2 = High Sodium   3 = High Refined Sugar   5 = Cholesterol
1+ = Very High Fat   2+ = Very High Sodium   4 = Highly Processed   ★= Better Choice

VARIETY *(Brand)*   RATING CODE

VARIETY (Brand)	★	1	2	3	4
Rice Cakes, Mini Plain *(Hain)*	★				
Rice Cakes, Mini Plain, No Salt *(Hain)*	★				
Rice Cakes, Mini Teriyaki *(Hain)*			2		
Rice Cakes, Mochi, Low Sodium *(Lundberg)*			2		
Rice Cakes, Multi-Grain *(Chico San)*	★				
Rice Cakes, Plain *(Hain)*	★				
Rice Cakes, Plain, No Salt Added *(Hain)*	★				
Rice Cakes, Plain, No Sodium *(Quaker)*	★				
Rice Cakes, Popcorn, Sodium Free *(Lundberg)*	★				
Rice Cakes, Sesame *(Hain)*	★				
Rice Cakes, Sesame, No Salt *(Hain)*	★				
Rice Cakes, Sesame Garlic *(Westbrae Natural)*			2		
Rice Cakes, Teriyaki *(Westbrae Natural)*	★				
Rice Cakes, Wehani, Low Sodium *(Lundberg)*			2		
Rice Cakes, Wild Rice, Low Sodium *(Lundberg)*			2		
Rye Cakes *(Quaker)*	★				
Sesame Cakes *(Quaker)*	★				
Sesame Cakes, No Sodium *(Quaker)*	★				
Sesame Crunch *(Barbara's)*		1+		3	
Sesame Oat Bran Sticks *(Good Sense)*		1	2		4
Snack Sticks, Pretzel *(Pepperidge Farm)*			2+		4
Snack Sticks, Pumpernickel *(Pepperidge Farm)*		1	2		4
Snack Sticks, Sesame *(Pepperidge Farm)*		1	2		4
Snack Sticks, Three Cheese *(Pepperidge Farm)*		1	2+		4
Teddy Grahams, Cinnamon *(Nabisco)*				3	4
Teddy Grahams, Honey *(Nabisco)*				3	4
Teddy Grahams, Vanilla *(Nabisco)*				3	4
Tortilla Chips *(Chi-Chi's)*		1+			
Tortilla Chips, Buenitos *(Health Valley)*		1			
Tortilla Chips, Buenitos, No Salt *(Health Valley)*		1			
Tortilla Chips, Cantina Style *(Frito Lay)*		1+			
Tortilla Chips, Restaurant Style *(Frito Lay)*		1+			
Tortilla Chips, Sesame *(Hain)*		1			

1 = High Fat   2 = High Sodium   3 = High Refined Sugar   5 = Cholesterol
1+ = Very High Fat   2+ = Very High Sodium   4 = Highly Processed   ★= Better Choice

VARIETY *(Brand)*   RATING CODE

Tortilla Chips, Sesame, No Salt *(Hain)*		1		
Tortilla Chips, Sesame Cheese *(Hain)*		1	2	
Vege Chips *(Edward & Sons)*	★			
Wheat Cakes *(Quaker)*			2	4
Wheat Cakes, Light Salt *(Konriko)*	★			
Wheat Cakes, No Salt *(Konriko)*	★			
Wheat Free Pastry Popper, Blueberry *(Natures Warehouse)*	★			
Wheat Free Pastry Popper, Cherry *(Natures Warehouse)*	★			
Wheat Free Pastry Popper, Peach Apricot *(Natures Warehouse)*	★			
Wheat Free Pastry Popper, Raspberry *(Natures Warehouse)*	★			
White Cheddar Popped Corn Cakes *(Quaker)*			2+	4

1 = High Fat	2 = High Sodium	3 = High Refined Sugar	5 = Cholesterol
1+ = Very High Fat	2+ = Very High Sodium	4 = Highly Processed	★= Better Choice

SOUPS

Grandma would always prepare soup when someone was ill. It was warm, comforting to the tummy and easy to digest. It had health written all over it. Today, to compete with the taste requirements of most Americans, salt has been added — and added abundantly. Fat has been added to the cream style soups, and additives and preservatives such as MSG, tropical oils, cottonseed oil, etc. are added. I had to omit many soups from *The Food Bible*, but I still feel that soup can be a good food choice. We just need to watch the sodium and really limit those with a (2+) rating code.

VARIETY *(Brand)*   RATING CODE

SOUPS
CANNED

Asparagus, Golden Classic *(Campbell's)*	1 2+		
Beef & Pasta Bordeaux Light Balance *(Lunch Bucket)*	2+	4	
Beef Americana, Light Balance *(Lunch Bucket)*	2+	4	5
Beef Barley *(Progresso)*	2+		5
Beef Minestrone *(Progresso)*	2+		
Beef Noodle *(Progresso)*	2+		
Beef Soup *(Progresso)*	1 2+		5
Beef Vegetable *(Progresso)*	2+		
Beef with Vegetables & Barley, Manhandler *(Campbell's)*	2+		
Black Bean *(Health Valley)*	2		
Black Bean, No Salt *(Health Valley)*	★		
Broth, Beef *(Health Valley)*	1+ 2+		
Broth, Beef *(Pritikin)*	2+		
Broth, Beef, No Salt *(Health Valley)*	1+		
Broth, Chicken *(Hain)*	1+ 2+		
Broth, Chicken *(Health Valley)*	1+ 2+		
Broth, Chicken *(Pritikin)*	1+ 2+		
Broth, Chicken *(Shelton's)*	1+ 2+		
Broth, Chicken, Low Fat & Low Sodium *(Shelton's)*	1+ 2		
Broth, Chicken, Low Sodium *(Campbell's)*	1+ 2		
Broth, Chicken, Natural Goodness, 1/3 Less Salt *(Swanson)*	1 2+		
Broth, Chicken, No Salt *(Health Valley)*	1+		
Broth, Chicken, No Salt Added *(Hain)*	1+		
Chicken Cacciatore, Light Balance *(Lunch Bucket)*	2+	4	5
Chicken Fiesta, Light Balance *(Lunch Bucket)*	2+	4	
Chicken Gumbo *(Pritikin)*	★		
Chicken Noodle *(Hain)*	2+		5
Chicken Noodle, No Salt Added *(Hain)*	1		5
Chicken Nuggets with Vegetables & Noodles, Chunky *(Campbell's)*	1 2+		
Chicken Rice, Home Cookin' *(Campbell's)*	1 2+	4	
Chicken Soup with Pasta *(Pritikin)*	2	4	
Chicken Vegetable *(Pritikin)*	2		
Chicken with Noodles, Low Sodium *(Campbell's)*		4	

---

1 = High Fat   2 = High Sodium   3 = High Refined Sugar   5 = Cholesterol
1+ = Very High Fat   2+ = Very High Sodium   4 = Highly Processed   ★= Better Choice

VARIETY (Brand)   RATING CODE

Variety (Brand)	★	Fat	Sodium	4	5
Chili Beef (Campbell's)			2+		
Chili Beef with Beans, Manhandler (Campbell's)		1	2+		
Clam Chowder, Manhattan (Health Valley)			2+		
Clam Chowder, Manhattan Style (Progresso)			2+		
Clam Chowder, Manhattan, No Salt (Health Valley)	★				
Clam Chowder, New England (Hain)			2+		5
Clam Chowder, New England (Pritikin)	★				
Clam Chowder, New England Style (Progresso)			2+		
Hearty Beef with Vegetables & Pasta, Home Cookin' (Campbell's)			2+		5
Italian Vege-Pasta (Hain)			2+		5
Italian Vege-Pasta, Low Sodium (Hain)		1			5
Lentil (Health Valley)			2		
Lentil (Pritikin)			2		
Lentil (Progresso)			2+		
Lentil (Victoria)			2+		
Lentil, No Salt (Health Valley)	★				
Macaroni & Bean (Progresso)			2+	4	
Minestrone (Hain)			2+		
Minestrone (Health Valley)			2+		
Minestrone (Pritikin)	★				
Minestrone (Victoria)			2+		
Minestrone, Italian Style (Progresso)			2+		
Minestrone, No Salt (Health Valley)	★				
Minestrone, No Salt Added (Hain)	★				
Minestrone, Original Recipe (Progresso)			2+		
Mushroom Barley (Hain)			2+		
Mushroom Barley (Health Valley)			2+		
Mushroom Barley, No Salt (Health Valley)	★				
Mushroom, Creamy (Hain)		1	2+		
Mushroom, No Salt (Health Valley)		1			
Pasta & Bean (Victoria)			2+	4	
Pasta & Garden Vegetables, Light Balance (Lunch Bucket)			2+	4	
Potato (Health Valley)	★				

1 = High Fat	2 = High Sodium	3 = High Refined Sugar	5 = Cholesterol
1+ = Very High Fat	2+ = Very High Sodium	4 = Highly Processed	★= Better Choice

VARIETY *(Brand)*   RATING CODE

Potato Leek *(Health Valley)*	2	
Potato Leek, No Salt *(Health Valley)*	★	
Potato, Creamy, Natural, Golden Classic *(Campbell's)*	1+ 2+	
Split Pea *(Hain)*	2+	
Split Pea *(Health Valley)*	★	
Split Pea *(Pritikin)*	★	
Split Pea, No Salt *(Health Valley)*	★	
Split Pea, No Salt Added *(Hain)*	★	
Tomato *(Health Valley)*	2+	
Tomato *(Town House)*	2+	
Tomato Garden, Home Cookin' *(Campbell's)*	2+	
Tomato with Vegetables & Macaroni *(Progresso)*	2+	
Tomato with Tomato Pieces *(Pritikin)*	2	
Tomato, Cream of - Homestyle *(Campbell's)*	2+	
Tomato, No Salt *(Health Valley)*	★	
Tomato, Zesty *(Campbell's)*	2+	
Turkey Rice *(Hain)*	2+	5
Turkey Rice, No Salt Added *(Hain)*		5
Turkey Vegetable with Pasta *(Pritikin)*	2+	
Vegetable *(Health Valley)*	2	
Vegetable *(Pritikin)*	2	
Vegetable *(Progresso)*	2+	
Vegetable Beef *(Campbell's)*	2+	
Vegetable Chicken *(Hain)*	2+	
Vegetable Chicken, No Salt Added *(Hain)*		5
Vegetable, Chunky Chicken *(Health Valley)*	2+	
Vegetable, Chunky Chicken, No Salt *(Health Valley)*	★	
Vegetable, Chunky Five Bean *(Health Valley)*	2+	
Vegetable, Chunky Five Bean, No Salt *(Health Valley)*	★	
Vegetable, No Salt *(Health Valley)*	★	
Vegetarian Lentil *(Hain)*	2+	
Vegetarian Lentil, No Salt Added *(Hain)*	★	
Vegetarian Vegetable *(Hain)*	2+	

---

1 = High Fat	2 = High Sodium	3 = High Refined Sugar	5 = Cholesterol
1+ = Very High Fat	2+ = Very High Sodium	4 = Highly Processed	★= Better Choice

VARIETY *(Brand)*   RATING CODE

Vegetarian Vegetable, No Salt Added *(Hain)*	★	
DRY MIXES		
Asparagus Mix *(Knorr)*	2+	
Beef Stew, Family Favorites Mix, Prepared with Lean Meat *(Lipton)*	2+	5
Cheddar, Creamy *(Fantastic Foods)*	1 2+	
Cheese & Broccoli Mix *(Hain)*	1+ 2+	
Cheese Soup & Sauce Mix *(Hain)*	1+ 2+	
Chicken Dijonnaise Mix *(Knorr)*	2+	
Chicken Noodle Mix *(Knorr)*	2+	
Chicken Noodle with White Meat - Cup *(Campbell's)*	2+	4
Chicken Style, Prepared *(Mayacamas)*	2+	
Clam Chowder, Prepared *(Mayacamas)*	2+	
Cockie Leekie *(Mayacamas)*	2+	
Coq au Vin Mix *(Knorr)*	2+	
Country Chicken, Family Favorite Mix, Prepared with Lean Meat *(Lipton)*	2+	5
French Onion Mix *(Knorr)*	2+	
French Onion, Prepared *(Mayacamas)*	2+	
Leek Mix *(Knorr)*	2+	
Lentil Mix *(Hain)*	2+	
Minestrone Mix *(Hain)*	2+	
Mushroom Mix *(Hain)*	1+ 2+	
Mushroom Mix, No Salt Added *(Hain)*	1+	
Noodle with Chicken Broth - Cup *(Campbell's)*	2+	4
Onion Soup & Dip Mix *(Hain)*	1 2+	
Onion Soup & Dip Mix, No Salt Added *(Hain)*	2+	
Oxtail Mix *(Knorr)*	2+	
Pea, Garden, Prepared *(Mayacamas)*	2+	
Potato Leek Mix *(Hain)*	1+ 2	
Spinach Mix *(Knorr)*	2+	
Split Pea Mix *(Hain)*	2+	
Tomato Mix *(Hain)*	1+ 2+	
Tomato with Basil Mix *(Knorr)*	2+	

VARIETY (*Brand*)   RATING CODE

Vegetable Mix *(Hain)*	2+
Vegetable Mix, No Salt Added *(Hain)*	2+
Vegetable, Curry *(Fantastic Foods)*	1 2+
Vegetable, Miso *(Fantastic Foods)*	1 2
Vegetable, Tomato *(Fantastic Foods)*	1 2
FROZEN	
Lentil *(Tabatchnick)*	2+
Minestrone *(Tabatchnick)*	2+
Vegetable *(Tabatchnick)*	2+

---

1 = High Fat	2 = High Sodium	3 = High Refined Sugar	5 = Cholesterol
1+ = Very High Fat	2+ = Very High Sodium	4 = Highly Processed	★= Better Choice

SPICES

Spices are great to use to give foods distinctive tastes without using salt. There are many good spices available which are mixtures of herbs; however, some contain MSG as well as other additives and preservatives. Let's look at a couple of spices that didn't make it in *The Food Bible*.

Durkee Sweet Pepper Flakes	sodium sulfite and sodium bisulfite
Lawry's Seasoning Salt	MSG

I have listed the spices a bit differently. It would be impractical to list all spices because there are so many. I'm giving you examples of spices without sodium and then examples of spices with sodium — of course, none contains additives or preservatives. Personally, I use spices without sodium.

VARIETY *(Brand)*   RATING CODE

SPICES
SPICES WITH SODIUM
Cajun Seasonings *(Chef Paul Prudhomme's)*   2+
Celery Salt *(Durkee)*   2+
Garlic Salt *(Spice Islands)*   2+

Lemon Pepper *(Lawry's)*   2+
Meat Tenderizer *(Adolph's)*   2+
Onion Salt *(McCormick)*   2+

Seasoned Salt *(Spice Classics)*   2+

SPICES WITHOUT SODIUM
All-Purpose Seasoning *(Tones)*   ★
Chicken & Fish Seasoning *(Natural Blend)*   ★
Crab, Crawfish & Shrimp Boil, Boxed *(Zatarain's)* ★

Instead of Salt *(Health Valley)*   ★
Mrs. Dash *(Mrs. Dash)*   ★
Mrs. Dash, Herb & Garlic *(Mrs. Dash)*   ★

Original Herb *(American Heart Assoc.)*   ★
Pepper, Seasoned *(Lawry's)*   ★
Sesame, All Purpose *(Parsley Patch)*   ★

Vegetable & Salad Seasoning *(Natural Blend)*   ★

SYRUPS

Most all syrups are high in refined sugar; however, there are a few that are made with fruit juice and no refined sugar. Also, most all brands of waffle and pancake syrups contain artificial flavor in addition to other additives. For example: *Aunt Jemima Lite* and *Log Cabin* both contain artificial flavors and sodium benzoate.

I don't use syrups often, but when I do, it will be a natural maple or a fruit syrup made without refined sugar. I will use molasses in cookies or muffins.

VARIETY *(Brand)*   RATING CODE

SYRUPS			
Apricot *(Knott's Berry Farm)*		3	4
Blackberry *(Knott's Berry Farm)*		3	4
Blackberry *(Smucker's)*		3	4
Blueberry *(Knott's Berry Farm)*		3	4
Blueberry *(R. W. Knudsen)*	★		
Blueberry *(Smucker's)*		3	4
Boysenberry *(Knott's Berry Farm)*		3	4
Boysenberry *(R. W. Knudsen)*	★		
Fruit 'n Maple *(R. W. Knudsen)*	★		
Maple Syrup *(Camp)*		3	4
Maple Syrup *(Cary's)*		3	4
Maple Syrup *(Spring Tree)*		3	4
Maple Syrup *(Vermont)*		3	4
Molasses, Black Strap *(Plantation)*		3	
Molasses, Black Strap *(Slow As)*		3	
Molasses, Light & Dark *(Brer Rabbit)*		3	
Molasses, Unsulfured *(Grandma's)*		3	
Molasses, Unsulphered *(New Morning)*		3	
Raspberry *(R. W. Knudsen)*	★		
Ribbon Cane Syrup *(Renfro's)*		3	4
Sorghum Molasses *(Hillbilly)*		3	4
Sorghum Molasses *(Ozarka)*		3	4
Sorghum Syrup & Molasses *(Renfro's)*		3	4
Strawberry *(Knott's Berry Farm)*		3	4
Strawberry *(R. W. Knudsen)*	★		
Strawberry *(Smucker's)*		3	4

VEGETABLES

Fresh, frozen or canned — is one better than another? No, not entirely. I feel that each has its strong points. For example: The legumes are certainly more convenient and equally nutritious when canned. I will have to say that I personally will choose fresh vegetables first when they're in season and when they look decent. Most vegetables are unlike fruit in that they can be picked prematurely and still taste good and retain most all their nutrients. A long truck ride from south Texas to Chicago is not going to effect the quality of fresh vegetables that much.

The important thing is that we include them in our diets, both the complex and simple carbohydrate types. Complex carbohydrates include potatoes, beans (legumes), peas, sweet potatoes, corn, and winter squash, while the simple carbohydrates include all the other vegetables. Practically all plain, canned and frozen vegetables are free of additives and preservatives. In fact, the only thing to watch is the salt that is added to canned and frozen vegetables. If you are watching your sodium, there are plenty of the salt-free vegetables from which to choose.

VARIETY *(Brand)*   RATING CODE

VEGETABLES
CANNED

Variety (Brand)	Rating Code
Artichoke Bottoms *(Fancifood)*	★
Artichoke Bottoms *(Gourmet Award)*	★
Artichoke Bottoms *(Reese)*	★
Artichoke Hearts *(Pope)*	★
Artichoke Hearts *(Progresso)*	★
Artichoke Hearts *(Roland)*	★
Artichoke Hearts *(S & W)*	★
Artichoke Hearts, Marinated *(Fancifood)*	1+
Artichoke Hearts, Marinated *(Progresso)*	1+ 2
Artichoke Hearts, Quartered *(Gourmet Award)*	★
Artichoke Hearts, Spanish *(Reese)*	★
Artichoke Hearts, Whole *(Gourmet Award)*	★
Artichoke Hearts, Whole *(South Shore)*	★
Asparagus *(Del Monte)*	2+
Asparagus *(Green Giant)*	2+
Asparagus *(Joan of Arc)*	2+
Asparagus *(Walla Walla)*	2+
Asparagus Spears *(Hokan)*	2+
Asparagus Spears *(Reese)*	2+
Asparagus Spears *(S & W)*	2+
Asparagus, Cut *(Thank You)*	2+
Asparagus, Tender Green *(Green Giant)*	2+
Asparagus, Tender Green *(Le Sueur)*	2+
Asparagus, White *(Gourmet Award)*	2+
Baby Corn, Pickled *(Hokan)*	2+
Beans, Great Northern *(Bush's)*	2+
Beans, Great Northern *(Green Giant)*	2+
Beans, Great Northern *(Rainbow)*	2+
Beans, Navy *(Bush's)*	2+
Beets *(Del Monte)*	2+ 3
Beets *(Libby's)*	2+ 3
Beets *(Rainbow)*	2+
Beets *(Town House)*	2+

VARIETY *(Brand)*   RATING CODE

Beets, Harvard *(Aunt Nellie's)*	2+ 3
Beets, Pickled *(Aunt Nellie's)*	2+ 3
Beets, Pickled *(Del Monte)*	2+ 3
Beets, Pickled with Onions *(Aunt Nellie's)*	2+ 3
Beets, Sliced *(ReNa)*	2
Beets, Whole *(S & W)*	2
Beets, Whole & Sliced *(Stokely's)*	2+
Butter Beans *(Bush's)*	2+
Cabbage, Red *(Aunt Nellie's)*	2+
Carrots *(Aunt Nellie's)*	2+
Carrots *(Ro-tel)*	2+
Carrots & Peas *(ReNa)*	2+
Carrots, Belgian *(ReNa)*	2+
Carrots, Crinkle Sliced *(Freshlike)*	2+
Carrots, Cut & Sliced *(Del Monte)*	2+
Carrots, Extra Tiny *(Reese)*	2+
Carrots, Fingerling *(Thank You)*	2+
Carrots, Julienne *(S & W)*	2+
Carrots, Sliced *(Allen's)*	2+
Carrots, Sliced *(Libby's)*	2+
Carrots, Sliced *(Stokely's)*	2+
Carrots, Tiny Whole *(S & W)*	2+
Collard Greens *(Allen's)*	2+
Corn, Cream Style *(Del Monte)*	2+
Corn, Cream Style *(Freshlike)*	2+
Corn, Cream Style *(Green Giant)*	2+
Corn, Cream Style *(Libby's)*	2+
Corn, Cream Style *(Mile High)*	2+
Corn, Cream Style *(S & W)*	2+
Corn, Cream Style *(Stokely's)*	2+
Corn, Cream Style *(Town House)*	2+
Corn, Cream Style, No Salt *(Del Monte)*	★
Corn, Dried *(John Copes)*	★

1 = High Fat	2 = High Sodium	3 = High Refined Sugar	5 = Cholesterol
1+ = Very High Fat	2+ = Very High Sodium	4 = Highly Processed	★= Better Choice

VARIETY *(Brand)*   RATING CODE

Corn, Mexicorn *(Green Giant)*	2+
Corn, Sweet Nibblets *(Green Giant)*	2
Corn, White *(Del Monte)*	2+
Corn, White *(Green Giant)*	2
Corn, White Shoe Peg *(Del Monte)*	2+
Corn, White, Cream Style *(Stokely's)* .	2+
Corn, Whole Baby *(China Bowl)*	2+
Corn, Whole Baby *(Gourmet Award)*	2
Corn, Whole Baby *(Reese)*	2
Corn, Whole Kernel *(Del Monte)*	2+
Corn, Whole Kernel *(Featherweight)*	★
Corn, Whole Kernel *(Green Giant)*	2
Corn, Whole Kernel *(Kounty Kist)*	2
Corn, Whole Kernel *(Libby's)*	2+
Corn, Whole Kernel *(Mile High)*	2
Corn, Whole Kernel *(Rainbow)*	2+
Corn, Whole Kernel *(Stokely's)*	2+
Corn, Whole Kernel *(Town House)*	2
Corn, Whole Kernel, Natural Pack *(Libby's)*	★
Corn, Whole Kernel, Low Salt *(Green Giant)*	2
Corn, Whole Kernel, No Salt *(Del Monte)*	★
Garden Medley *(Green Giant)*	2+
Garden Salad *(Read)*	2+ 3
Garden Salad *(ReNa)*	2+
Garden Salad, Dill *(S & W)*	2+
Green Beans *(Mile High)*	2+
Green Beans *(ReNa)*	2+
Green Beans *(S & W)*	2+
Green Beans and Shellouts *(Allen's)*	2+
Green Beans and Shelly Beans *(Bush's)*	2+
Green Beans, Almondine *(Green Giant)*	2+
Green Beans, Cut *(Freshlike)*	2+
Green Beans, Cut *(Green Giant)*	2+

VARIETY *(Brand)*   RATING CODE

Variety (Brand)	Rating
Green Beans, Cut *(Libby's)*	2+
Green Beans, Cut and Whole *(Stokely's)*	2+
Green Beans, Cut, Low Salt *(Green Giant)*	★
Green Beans, Cut, No Salt *(Del Monte)*	★
Green Beans, Cut, Whole & French Style *(Del Monte)*	2+
Green Beans, Cut, Whole & French Style *(Town House)*	2+
Green Beans, French Style *(Freshlike)*	2+
Green Beans, French Style *(Green Giant)*	2+
Green Beans, French Style *(Libby's)*	2+
Green Beans, French Style *(Stokely's)*	2+
Green Beans, French Style, No Salt *(Del Monte)*	★
Green Beans, Italian *(Allen's)*	2+
Green Beans, Italian *(Del Monte)*	2+
Green Beans, Regular Cut *(Rainbow)*	2+
Green Beans, Seasoned *(Allen's)*	2+
Green Beans, Seasoned *(Del Monte)*	2+
Green Beans, Seeds Only *(ReNa)*	2+
Green Beans, Sliced *(Kounty Kist)*	2+
Green Beans, Whole *(B & B)*	2+
Green Beans, Whole *(S & W)*	2+
Hominy *(Milpas)*	2+
Hominy, Mexican Style *(Juanita's)*	2+
Kraut *(Del Monte)*	2+
Kraut, Bavarian *(Bush's)*	2+
Kraut, Chopped & Shredded *(Bush's)*	2+
Kraut, Ko-Mic *(New Morning)*	2+
Lima Beans *(Allen's)*	2+
Lima Beans *(Del Monte)*	2+
Mixed Greens *(Bush's)*	2+
Mixed Vegetables *(Del Monte)*	2+
Mixed Vegetables *(ReNa)*	2+
Mixed Vegetables *(Stokely's)*	2+
Mixed Vegetables *(Town House)*	2+

1 = High Fat   2 = High Sodium   3 = High Refined Sugar   5 = Cholesterol
1+ = Very High Fat   2+ = Very High Sodium   4 = Highly Processed   ★ = Better Choice

VARIETY *(Brand)*   RATING CODE

Variety (Brand)	Better Choice	Rating
Mixed Vegetables *(Veg-all)*		2+
Mixed Vegetables, Homestyle *(Veg-all)*		2+
Mixed Vegetables, Lite *(Veg-all)*	★	
Mushrooms *(Green Giant)*		2+
Mushrooms, Boiled in Butter *(Green Giant)*		1 2+
Mushrooms, Broiled in Butter *(B & B)*		1 2+
Mushrooms, Buttons, Slices, Pieces & Stems *(Giorgio)*		2+
Mushrooms, Buttons, Slices, Pieces & Stems *(Town House)*		2+
Mushrooms, No Salt *(Del Monte)*	★	
Mushrooms, Pieces & Stems *(Fancifood)*		2+
Mushrooms, Pieces & Stems *(Rainbow)*		2+
Mushrooms, Sliced *(Green Giant)*		2+
Mushrooms, Sliced, Pieces & Stems *(Gourmet Award)*		2+
Mushrooms, Stems & Pieces *(Brandywine)*		2+
Mushrooms, Stems & Pieces *(Pennsylvania Dutchman)*		2+
Mushrooms, Straw *(Green Giant)*		2+
Okra & Tomatoes *(Bush's)*		2+
Okra & Tomatoes *(Trappey's)*		2+
Okra, Cut *(Trappey's)*		2+
Olive Appetizer *(Progresso)*		1+ 2+
Olive Salad *(Progresso)*		1+ 2+
Onions, White *(ReNa)*		2+
Onions, Whole *(S & W)*		2+
Onions, Whole *(Thank You)*		2+
Peas *(Del Monte)*		2+
Peas *(Green Giant)*		2+
Peas *(Le Sueur)*		2+
Peas *(Libby's)*		2+
Peas *(Lindy)*		2+
Peas *(Mile High)*		2+
Peas *(Rainbow)*		2+
Peas *(ReNa)*		2+
Peas *(S & W)*		2+

VARIETY *(Brand)*   RATING CODE

Variety (Brand)	Better Choice	Rating
Peas *(Stokely's)*		2+
Peas *(Town House)*		2+
Peas and Carrots *(Del Monte)*	★	
Peas and Carrots *(Veg-all)*	★	
Peas and Onions *(Green Giant)*		2+
Peas and Onions *(S & W)*		2+
Peas, Blended Sweet *(Featherweight)*	★	
Peas, Crowder *(Griffin's)*		2+
Peas, Early June *(Kounty Kist)*		2+
Peas, Green *(Aunt Nellie's)*		2+
Peas, Green, No Salt *(Del Monte)*	★	
Peas, Low Salt *(Green Giant)*	★	
Peas, Mexican Style *(ReNa)*		2+
Peas, Natural Pack *(Libby's)*	★	
Peppers, Roasted Red Bell *(Mezzetta)*		2+
Pimientos *(Goya)*	★	
Pimientos, Diced & Sliced *(Dromedary)*	★	
Pimientos, Sliced & Diced *(O-Sage)*	★	
Potatoes *(Del Monte)*		2+
Potatoes *(ReNa)*		2+
Red Cabbage, Sweet-Sour *(Greenwood)*		2+ 3
Sauerkraut *(Cosmic)*		2+
Sauerkraut *(Del Monte)*		2+
Sauerkraut *(Eden)*		2+
Sauerkraut *(Libby's)*		2+
Sauerkraut *(Silver Floss)*		2+
Sauerkraut *(Town House)*		2+
Sauerkraut, Chopped *(Stokely's)*		2+
Sauerkraut, Low Sodium *(Cascadian Farm)*		2+
Sauerkraut, Low Sodium *(New Morning)*		2+
Sauerkraut, Shredded *(Stokely's)*		2+
Sauerkraut, Specialities *(Del Monte)*		2+
Shellie Beans *(Stokely's)*		2+

VARIETY *(Brand)*   RATING CODE

Spinach *(Bush's)*	2+
Spinach *(Del Monte)*	2+
Spinach *(Rainbow)*	2+
Spinach *(ReNa)*	2+
Spinach *(Stokely's)*	2+
Spinach, No Salt *(Del Monte)*	2+
Spinach, Popeye *(Allen's)*	2+
Spinach, Whole Leaf *(Town House)*	2+
Spinach, Whole Leaf, No Salt *(Del Monte)*	2+
Sweet Potatoes *(Taylor's)*	3
Three Bean Salad *(Green Giant)*	2+
Three Bean Salad *(Read)*	2+ 3
Tomatoes *(Gardenside)*	2+
Tomatoes *(Kruner's)*	2+
Tomatoes *(Mile High)*	2+
Tomatoes *(Progresso)*	2+
Tomatoes *(Rainbow)*	2+
Tomatoes *(Ro-tel)*	2+
Tomatoes in Tomato Juice *(Del Monte)*	2+
Tomatoes with Green Chilies *(Ashley's)*	2+
Tomatoes with Green Chilies *(Ro-tel)*	2+
Tomatoes with Jalapeños *(Contadina)*	2+
Tomatoes with Okra *(Superfine)*	2+
Tomatoes with Peels *(Del Monte)*	2+
Tomatoes, Aspic *(Reese)*	2+
Tomatoes, Aspic *(S & W)*	2+
Tomatoes, Cajun Stewed *(Del Monte)*	2+
Tomatoes, Cajun Style, Stewed *(S & W)*	2+
Tomatoes, Crushed *(Progresso)*	2+
Tomatoes, Diced *(Del Monte)*	2+
Tomatoes, Italian Crushed, Stewed & Whole *(Hunt's)*	2+
Tomatoes, Italian Stewed *(Del Monte)*	2+
Tomatoes, Italian Style, Stewed *(S & W)*	2+

VARIETY *(Brand)*   RATING CODE

Variety (Brand)		Rating
Tomatoes, Mexican Stewed *(Del Monte)*		2+
Tomatoes, Mexican Style, Stewed *(S & W)*		2+
Tomatoes, No Salt *(Hunt's)*	★	
Tomatoes, Peeled & Ready Cut *(S & W)*		2+
Tomatoes, Peeled, Italian with Basil *(Progresso)*		2+
Tomatoes, Redi-cut *(Hunt's)*		2+
Tomatoes, Stewed *(Contadina)*		2+
Tomatoes, Stewed *(Del Monte)*		2+
Tomatoes, Stewed *(S & W)*		2+
Tomatoes, Stewed *(Stokely's)*		2+
Tomatoes, Stewed *(Town House)*		2+
Tomatoes, Stewed, Chunky, Pasta Style *(Del Monte)*		2+
Tomatoes, Stewed, No Salt *(Del Monte)*	★	
Tomatoes, Stewed, No Salt *(Hunt's)*	★	
Tomatoes, Wedges *(Del Monte)*		2+
Tomatoes, Whole *(Contadina)*		2+
Tomatoes, Whole *(Del Monte)*		2+
Tomatoes, Whole *(Ro-tel)*		2+
Tomatoes, Whole *(Stokely's)*		2+
Tomatoes, Whole *(Town House)*		2+
Tomatoes, Whole, No Salt *(Hunt's)*	★	
Turnip Greens with Diced Turnips *(Bush's)*		2+
Wax Beans, Cut *(Del Monte)*		2+
Yams *(Allen's)*		3
Yams *(Louisiana)*		3
Yams *(Princella)*		3
Yams *(Trappey's)*		3
Yams in Syrup *(Bruce's)*		3
Yams, Candied *(S & W)*		3
Yams, Golden *(Trappey's)*		3
Yams, Light Syrup *(Princella)*		3
Zucchini, Italian Style *(Del Monte)*		2+
Zucchini, Italian Style *(S & W)*		2+

VARIETY *(Brand)*   RATING CODE

FROZEN			
Asparagus Spears *(Bel-air)*	★		
Asparagus Spears *(Birds Eye)*	★		
Asparagus Spears *(VIP)*	★		
Asparagus Spears, Micro *(Bel-air)*	★		
Blackeyed Peas *(Bel-air)*	★		
Blackeyed Peas *(Stilwell)*	★		
Blackeyed Peas *(VIP)*	★		
Broccoli *(Freshlike)*	★		
Broccoli *(Health Valley)*	★		
Broccoli *(Pictsweet)*	★		
Broccoli *(VIP)*	★		
Broccoli and Cauliflower, Singles *(Stokely's)*	★		
Broccoli Carrot Fanfare *(Green Giant)*	★		
Broccoli Cuts *(Bel-air)*	★		
Broccoli Cuts *(Birds Eye)*	★		
Broccoli Cuts *(Green Giant)*	★		
Broccoli Cuts and Spears *(Stilwell)*	★		
Broccoli Spears *(Birds Eye)*	★		
Broccoli, Baby Carrots, Water Chestnuts *(Birds Eye)*	★		
Broccoli, Carrots, Cauliflower *(Birds Eye)*	★		
Brooooli, Carrots, Cauliflower *(Pictsweet)*	★		
Broccoli, Carrots, Water Chestnuts *(Bel-air)*	★		
Broccoli, Cauliflower *(Pictsweet)*	★		
Broccoli, Cauliflower *(Stilwell)*	★		
Broccoli, Cauliflower & Baby Whole Carrots *(Stokely's)*	★		
Broccoli, Cauliflower Supreme *(Green Giant)*		2	
Broccoli, Chopped *(Birds Eye)*	★		
Broccoli, Chopped & Spears *(Bel-air)*	★		
Broccoli, Corn, Red Peppers *(Birds Eye)*	★		
Broccoli, Corn, Red Peppers *(Pictsweet)*	★		
Broccoli, Cut & Spears, Harvest Fresh *(Green Giant)*		2+	
Broccoli, Japanese Style Vegetables *(Bel-air)*	★		
Broccoli, Red Peppers, Bamboo Shoots & Mushrooms *(Birds Eye)*	★		

1 = High Fat	2 = High Sodium	3 = High Refined Sugar	5 = Cholesterol
1+ = Very High Fat	2+ = Very High Sodium	4 = Highly Processed	★= Better Choice

VARIETY *(Brand)*	RATING CODE
Broccoli, Singles *(Stokely's)*	★
Brussel Sprouts *(Bel-air)*	★
Brussel Sprouts *(Freshlike)*	★
Brussel Sprouts *(Stilwell)*	★
Brussel Sprouts *(VIP)*	★
Brussel Sprouts, Express *(Pictsweet)*	★
California Mix *(VIP)*	★
California Style Vegetables *(Bel-air)*	★
California Style, American Mixture *(Green Giant)*	2
Capri *(Freshlike)*	4
Carrots, Baby *(Bel-air)*	★
Carrots, Baby *(Birds Eye)*	★
Carrots, Baby *(Stilwell)*	★
Carrots, Baby *(VIP)*	★
Carrots, Crinkle Cut *(Bel-air)*	★
Carrots, Crinkle Cut *(Stilwell)*	★
Carrots, Sliced *(Pictsweet)*	★
Carrots, Whole Baby *(Stokely's)*	★
Carrots, Whole Baby, Micro *(Birds Eye)*	★
Cauliflower *(Bel-air)*	★
Cauliflower *(Freshlike)*	★
Cauliflower *(Pictsweet)*	★
Cauliflower Florets *(Green Giant)*	★
Cauliflower, Baby Whole Carrots & Snow Pea Pods *(Birds Eye)*	★
Chinese Pea Pods *(Bel-air)*	★
Collards, Chopped *(Stilwell)*	★
Corn in Butter Sauce *(Freshlike)*	2
Corn Niblets, Harvest Fresh *(Green Giant)*	★
Corn, Baby Cob, Micro Pouch *(Birds Eye)*	★
Corn, Cut *(Stilwell)*	★
Corn, Cut *(VIP)*	★
Corn, Fiesta *(VIP)*	★
Corn, Nibblets *(Green Giant)*	★

1 = High Fat	2 = High Sodium	3 = High Refined Sugar	5 = Cholesterol
1+ = Very High Fat	2+ = Very High Sodium	4 = Highly Processed	★= Better Choice

VARIETY *(Brand)*   RATING CODE

Variety (Brand)	★				
Corn, Singles *(Stokely's)*	★				
Corn, Whole Kernel *(Bel-air)*	★				
Corn, Whole Kernel *(Freshlike)*	★				
Corn, Whole Kernel *(Health Valley)*	★				
Corn, Whole Kernel *(Pictsweet)*	★				
Corn, Whole Kernel Deluxe *(Birds Eye)*	★				
Corn-on-the-Cob *(Bel-air)*	★				
Corn-on-the-Cob *(Pictsweet)*	★				
Corn-on-the-Cob *(VIP)*	★				
Corn-on-the-Cob & Little Ears *(Birds Eye)*	★				
Corn-on-the-Cob, Mini Gold *(Ore-Ida)*	★				
Corn-on-the-Cob, Nibblers & Nibblet Ears *(Green Giant)*	★				
Corn-on-the-Cob, One Serving *(Green Giant)*	★				
Country Style Vegetables, Micro *(Bel-air)*	★				
Del Sol *(Freshlike)*				4	
Franciscan Vegetables *(VIP)*	★				
French Beans with Almonds, Express *(Pictsweet)*	★				
Fries, Long Branch Western Flavor *(Inland Valley)*		1	2		
Green Beans *(Freshlike)*	★				
Green Beans *(Health Valley)*	★				
Green Beans *(Stilwell)*	★				
Green Beans, Cut *(Birds Eye)*	★				
Green Beans, Cut & French Style *(VIP)*	★				
Green Beans, Cut, French Style & Italian *(Bel-air)*	★				
Green Beans, Harvest Fresh *(Green Giant)*			2+		
Green Peppers, Chopped *(Pictsweet)*	★				
Gumbo *(VIP)*	★				
Gumbo, Vegetable *(Stilwell)*	★				
Heartland Style, American Mixture *(Green Giant)*	★				
Italian Style Vegetable Combination *(VIP)*	★				
Italian Style Vegetables *(Bel-air)*	★				
Italian Style Vegetables *(VIP)*	★				
Japanese Vegetables *(Pictsweet)*	★				

1 = High Fat   2 = High Sodium   3 = High Refined Sugar   5 = Cholesterol
1+ = Very High Fat   2+ = Very High Sodium   4 = Highly Processed   ★ = Better Choice

VARIETY *(Brand)*   RATING CODE

Variety (Brand)	★			
Lima Beans *(Health Valley)*	★			
Lima Beans, Baby *(Bel-air)*	★			
Lima Beans, Baby *(Freshlike)*	★			
Lima Beans, Baby *(VIP)*	★			
Lima Beans, Fordhook *(Bel-air)*	★			
Lima Beans, Fordhook *(Freshlike)*	★			
Lima Beans, Harvest Fresh *(Green Giant)*		2		
Mandarin Stir-Fry Vegetables *(VIP)*	★			
Midwestern Blend *(Freshlike)*	★			
Milano *(Freshlike)*				4
Mixed Vegetables *(Birds Eye)*	★			
Mixed Vegetables *(Freshlike)*	★			
Mixed Vegetables *(Green Giant)*	★			
Mixed Vegetables *(Health Valley)*	★			
Mixed Vegetables *(Pictsweet)*	★			
Mixed Vegetables *(Stilwell)*	★			
Mixed Vegetables *(VIP)*	★			
Mixed Vegetables, Harvest Fresh *(Green Giant)*		2		
Mustard Greens *(Stilwell)*	★			
New England Style, American Mixture *(Green Giant)*	★			
Okra *(Pictsweet)*	★			
Okra *(VIP)*	★			
Okra, Cut *(Bel-air)*	★			
Okra, Tomatoes *(Pictsweet)*	★			
Okra, Whole *(Stilwell)*	★			
Okra, Whole, Express *(Pictsweet)*	★			
Old-Fashioned Vegetable Soup *(Pictsweet)*	★			
Onions, Chopped *(Bel-air)*	★			
Onions, Chopped *(Pictsweet)*	★			
Onions, Small in Cream Sauce *(Birds Eye)*		2+		
Oriental Vegetables *(VIP)*	★			
Peas *(Bel-air)*	★			
Peas *(Birds Eye)*		2		

1 = High Fat	2 = High Sodium	3 = High Refined Sugar	5 = Cholesterol
1+ = Very High Fat	2+ = Very High Sodium	4 = Highly Processed	★ = Better Choice

VARIETY *(Brand)* RATING CODE

Variety (Brand)				
Peas *(Freshlike)*	★			
Peas *(Green Giant)*		2		
Peas *(Health Valley)*	★			
Peas *(Pictsweet)*		2		
Peas *(Stilwell)*		2		
Peas *(VIP)*	★			
Peas and Carrots *(Bel-air)*	★			
Peas and Carrots *(Stilwell)*	★			
Peas and Carrots *(VIP)*	★			
Peas and Pearl Onions, Classic Mixtures, Micro *(Birds Eye)*	★			
Peas in Butter Sauce *(Freshlike)*		2+		
Peas, Baby Early, Harvest Fresh *(Green Giant)*		2		
Peas, Deluxe Snap, Micro *(Birds Eye)*	★			
Peas, Field with Snaps *(Pictsweet)*	★			
Peas, Sugar Snap, Micro *(Green Giant)*	★			
Peas, Sweet in Butter Sauce *(Birds Eye)*		1+	3	
Peas, Sweet, Harvest Fresh *(Green Giant)*		2		
Peking Stir-Fry Vegetables *(VIP)*	★			
Potato Chunks *(Mr. Dell's)*	★			
Potatoes, Curley Q Fries *(Inland Valley)*		1		
Potatoes, French Fries *(Ore Ida)*		1		
Potatoes, Golden Crinkles *(Ore-Ida)*		1		
Potatoes, Golden Fries *(Ore-Ida)*		1		
Potatoes, Golden Twirls *(Ore-Ida)*		1		
Potatoes, Hash Browns *(Ore-Ida)*	★			
Potatoes, O'Brien *(Bel-air)*	★			
Potatoes, O'Brien *(Ore-Ida)*	★			
Potatoes, Pixie Crinkles *(Ore-Ida)*		1+		
Potatoes, Shoestring *(Ore-Ida)*		1		
Primavera *(Freshlike)*			4	
Rancho Fiesta Style Vegetables, Micro *(Bel-air)*		2		
Rice, French Style *(Birds Eye)*		2	4	
Rice, Peas, Mushrooms *(Green Giant)*		2+	4	

1 = High Fat 2 = High Sodium 3 = High Refined Sugar 5 = Cholesterol
1+ = Very High Fat 2+ = Very High Sodium 4 = Highly Processed ★= Better Choice

VARIETY *(Brand)*   RATING CODE

VARIETY (Brand)	★	1	2	2+	5
Rotini Cheddar, Garden Gourmet *(Green Giant)*			2		
San Francisco Style, American Mixture *(Green Giant)*	★				
Santa Fe Style, American Mixture *(Green Giant)*	★				
Scandinavian Vegetables *(VIP)*	★				
Seasoning Blend, Chopped Onions *(Pictsweet)*	★				
Seasoning Vegetables *(Pictsweet)*	★				
Seattle Style, American Mixture *(Green Giant)*	★				
Shrimp Gumbo Mix *(Stilwell)*				2+	5
Snow Peas *(La Choy)*	★				
Spinach *(Freshlike)*	★				
Spinach *(Stilwell)*	★				
Spinach *(VIP)*	★				
Spinach, Cut Leaf *(Bel-air)*	★				
Spinach, Cut Leaf, Express *(Pictsweet)*	★				
Spinach, Harvest Fresh *(Green Giant)*				2+	
Squash, Yellow *(Pictsweet)*	★				
Stew Vegetables *(Bel-air)*	★				
Stew Vegetables *(Stilwell)*	★				
Stew Vegetables *(VIP)*	★				
Stir Fry, Japanese Style *(Birds Eye)*				2+	
Tator Babies, Western Spicy *(Inland Valley)*		1			
Turnip Greens, Chopped with Diced Turnips *(VIP)*			2		
Vegetable Soup Mix *(Stilwell)*				2+	
Vegetables for Stew *(Freshlike)*	★				
Winter Mix, Micro *(Bel-air)*	★				
Wisconsin Blend *(Freshlike)*	★				

1 = High Fat	2 = High Sodium	3 = High Refined Sugar	5 = Cholesterol
1+ = Very High Fat	2+ = Very High Sodium	4 = Highly Processed	★= Better Choice

VINEGAR

Vinegar can certainly add zip and create an interesting dish. Different vinegars are fun to use when looking for a new taste. Sometimes I will make a salad dressing using an herb vinegar, then add some of my own spices as well as a garlic clove.

Some wine vinegars contain sulfites as well as other additives and preservatives. As an example: *Heinz* Gourmet Wine Vinegar contains sulfur dioxide. Choose only these listed in *The Food Bible.*

VARIETY *(Brand)*   RATING CODE

VINEGAR

Variety (Brand)	Rating Code
Apple Cider Vinegar *(Eden)*	★
Apple Cider Vinegar *(Garden Club)*	★
Apple Cider Vinegar *(Heinz)*	2+
Apple Cider Vinegar *(New Morning)*	★
Apple Cider Vinegar *(Town House)*	★
Apple Cider Vinegar, Raw Unpasturized *(Hain)*	★
Blueberry Vinegar *(Rothschild)*	★
Cider Vinegar *(Hain)*	★
Fish 'n Chips Vinegar *(S & W)*	★
Garlic Vinegar *(Bertolli)*	★
Gourmet Vinegar, Malt *(Heinz)*	★
Gourmet Vinegar, Salad *(Heinz)*	★
Gourmet Vinegar, Tarragon *(Heinz)*	★
Herb Vinegar *(Paula's)*	★
Italian Garden Vinegar *(Paula's)*	★
Malt Vinegar *(Gourmet Award)*	★
Malt Vinegar *(Heinz)*	2+
Perfect Vinegar *(Paula's)*	★
Raspberry Royal Vinegar *(Paula's)*	★
Red Raspberry Vinegar *(Rothschild)*	★
Red Vinegar *(Bertolli)*	★
Rice Vinegar *(Gourmet Award)*	★
Rice Vinegar, Natural *(Nakano)*	★
Rice Vinegar, Two Chive *(Paula's)*	★
Salad Vinegar *(Heinz)*	2+
White Vinegar *(Bertolli)*	★
White Vinegar *(Garden Club)*	★
White Vinegar *(Heinz)*	2+
White Vinegar *(Rainbow)*	★
White Vinegar *(Town House)*	★
White Vinegar, Tarragon *(Gourmet Award)*	★

YOGURT

Yogurt can be a wonderfully nutritious food if we choose wisely. Many varieties of yogurt are sweetened with Nutra-Sweet or refined sugars, and some contain artificial flavors and artificial colors. Choose these listed below.

Yogurt is one of my favorite foods, and I eat it in a variety of ways. I make yogurt cheese by straining the whey from nonfat plain yogurt, then I spread it like cream cheese on a whole wheat bagel or whole wheat toast. I save the whey to use in pancakes or waffles. This gives them a light texture and a great flavor. For a wonderful snack, I add a little all-fruit jam, some fresh fruit and wheat germ to plain nonfat yogurt.

VARIETY *(Brand)*   **RATING CODE**

YOGURT
Apple Crisp *(New Country)* ... 3
Apricot, Lowfat *(Lucerne)* ... 3
Apricot Pineapple, Lowfat *(Lucerne)* ... 3

Awesome Peach, Nonrefrigerated *(Del Monte)* ... 3
Banana, Custard Style *(Yoplait)* ... 3 5
Banana, Original *(Dannon)* ... 3 5

Berries, Lowfat Breakfast *(Yoplait)* ... 3
Black Cherry *(Alta•Dena)* ... 3
Black Cherry *(Breyers)* ... 3

Black Cherry, Nonfat *(Alta•Dena)* ... ★
Blueberry *(Alta•Dena)* ... 3
Blueberry *(Breyers)* ... 3

Blueberry, Lowfat *(Alta•Dena)* ... 3
Blueberry, Lowfat *(Lucerne)* ... 3
Blueberry, Lowfat *(New Country)* ... 3

Blueberry, Lowfat Breakfast *(Dannon)* ... 3
Blueberry, Lowfat Original *(Yoplait)* ... 3
Blueberry, Nonfat *(Lucerne)* ... 3

Blueberry, Original *(Dannon)* ... 3 5
Boysenberry, Lowfat *(Lucerne)* ... 3
Boysenberry, Original *(Dannon)* ... 3 5

Caramel Pecan, Lowfat *(Lucerne)* ... 3
Cherry Supreme *(New Country)* ... 3
Cherry, Custard Style *(Yoplait)* ... 3

Cherry, Lowfat *(Lucerne)* ... 3
Cherry, Nonfat *(Lucerne)* ... 3
Cherry, Original *(Dannon)* ... 3 5

Dutch Apple, Original *(Dannon)* ... 3 5
Exotic Fruit, Original *(Dannon)* ... 3 5
Exotic Fruit, Original Lowfat *(Dannon)* ... 3

French Vanilla *(New Country)* ... 3
Fruit Crunch *(New Country)* ... 3
Hawaiian Salad *(New Country)* ... 3

1 = High Fat   2 = High Sodium   3 = High Refined Sugar   5 = Cholesterol
1+ = Very High Fat   2+ = Very High Sodium   4 = Highly Processed   ★= Better Choice

VARIETY *(Brand)* — RATING CODE

Variety (Brand)	Better Choice	Rating	
Lemon *(Alta·Dena)*		3	
Lemon *(New Country)*		3	
Lemon, Custard Style *(Yoplait)*		3	5
Lemon, Lowfat *(Lucerne)*		3	
Lemon, Lowfat Original *(Dannon)*		3	
Lemon, Lowfat Original *(Yoplait)*		3	
Lemon, Nonfat *(Weight Watchers)*		3	
Mixed Berries, Nonfat *(Alta·Dena)*	★		
Mixed Berries, Original Lowfat *(Dannon)*		3	
Mixed Berry *(Breyers)*		3	
Mixed Berry, Lowfat Original *(Yoplait)*		3	
Mixed Berry, Nonfat *(Weight Watchers)*		3	
Mixed Berry, Original *(Dannon)*		3	5
Orange, Lowfat *(Lucerne)*		3	
Peach *(Alta·Dena)*		3	
Peach *(Breyers)*		3	
Peach, Lowfat *(Lucerne)*		3	
Peach, Nonfat *(Alta·Dena)*	★		
Peach, Nonfat *(Lucerne)*		3	
Peach, Nonfat *(Weight Watchers)*		3	
Peach, Original *(Dannon)*		3	5
Piña Colada, Lowfat *(Lucerne)*		3	
Piña Colada, Lowfat Original *(Yoplait)*		3	
Piña Colada, Nonfat *(Alta·Dena)*	★		
Piña Colada, Original *(Dannon)*		3	5
Piña Colada, Original Lowfat *(Dannon)*		3	
Pineapple, Lowfat *(Alta·Dena)*		3	
Pineapple, Lowfat *(Lucerne)*		3	
Pineapple, Original Lowfat *(Dannon)*		3	
Plain, Lowfat *(Alta·Dena)*	★		
Plain, Lowfat *(Dannon)*	★		
Plain, Lowfat *(Lucerne)*	★		
Plain, Lowfat Original *(Yoplait)*	★		

1 = High Fat 1+ = Very High Fat 2 = High Sodium 2+ = Very High Sodium 3 = High Refined Sugar 4 = Highly Processed 5 = Cholesterol ★ = Better Choice

VARIETY *(Brand)*   RATING CODE

VARIETY (Brand)					
Plain, Maya *(Alta•Dena)*		1			
Plain, Nonfat *(Alta•Dena)*			2		
Plain, Nonfat *(Dannon)*	★				
Plain, Nonfat *(Lucerne)*	★				
Plain, Nonfat *(Weight Watchers)*	★				
Plain, Nonfat *(Yoplait)*				3	
Plain, Original Lowfat *(Dannon)*				3	
Raspberry Supreme *(New Country)*				3	
Raspberry, Custard Style *(Yoplait)*				3	5
Raspberry, Nonfat *(Weight Watchers)*				3	
Raspberry, Original *(Dannon)*				3	5
Red Raspberry *(Breyers)*				3	
Red Raspberry, Lowfat *(Alta•Dena)*				3	
Red Raspberry, Lowfat *(Lucerne)*				3	
Spiced Apple, Lowfat *(Lucerne)*				3	
Strawberry *(Alta•Dena)*				3	
Strawberry *(Breyers)*				3	
Strawberry *(New Country)*				3	
Strawberry Banana *(Breyers)*				3	
Strawberry Banana, Custard Style *(Yoplait)*				3	5
Strawberry Banana, Lowfat *(Lucerne)*				3	
Strawberry Banana, Nonfat *(Alta•Dena)*	★				
Strawberry Banana, Original *(Dannon)*				3	5
Strawberry, Custard Style *(Yoplait)*				3	5
Strawberry, Lowfat *(Lucerne)*				3	
Strawberry, Nonfat *(Alta•Dena)*	★				
Strawberry, Nonfat *(Lucerne)*				3	
Strawberry, Nonfat *(Weight Watchers)*				3	
Strawberry, Original *(Dannon)*				3	
Tropical Fruit, Lowfat Breakfast *(Yoplait)*				3	
Vanilla, Custard Style *(Yoplait)*				3	
Vanilla, Lowfat *(Alta•Dena)*				3	
Vanilla, Lowfat *(Lucerne)*				3	

1 = High Fat   2 = High Sodium   3 = High Refined Sugar   5 = Cholesterol
1+ = Very High Fat   2+ = Very High Sodium   4 = Highly Processed   ★= Better Choice

VARIETY *(Brand)*   RATING CODE

Vanilla, Lowfat Original *(Dannon)*		3
Vanilla, Nonfat *(Alta•Dena)*	★	
Vanilla, Nonfat *(Yoplait)*		3
Yogurt Split, Lowfat *(Lucerne)*		3

FOOD INDEX

356

Tofu, 269
Tofu Cookies, 163
Tofu Dinners and Side Dishes,
    184, 188, 269
Tomato Paste, 297
Tomato Sauce, 297-298
Tortellini Dinners and
    Side Dishes, 184, 188-189
Tortilla Chips, 249, 311-312
Tortilla Mix, 109
Tortillas, 249
Tostada Shells, 249
Tuna, 178, 238-239, 241
    Canned, 178, 238-239
        Oil Packed, 238
        Water Packed, 178, 238-239
    Frozen, 241
Turkey, 239, 241-242
Turkey Dinners and Entrées,
    181-182, 188-189
    Boxed and Canned, 181-182
    Frozen, 188
    Refrigerated, 189

—V—

Veal, 188, 241
Vegetable Oil, 261-263, 267-268
Vegetables, 177-178, 331-344
    Canned, 177-178, 331-338
    Dried, 332
    Frozen, 339-344
    Pickled, 157, 331-332
Vegetarian Dinners and Side Dishes,
    181-189
Vinegar, 269, 347

—W—

Waffle Mixes, 273
Walnuts, 258
Water Chestnuts, 269-270
Wheat Cakes, 312
Wheat Germ, 140
Whipping Cream, 253
White Sauce, 298
Wieners, 242
Worcestershire Sauce, 155

—Y—

Yogurt, 351-354
Yogurt, Frozen, 203-204

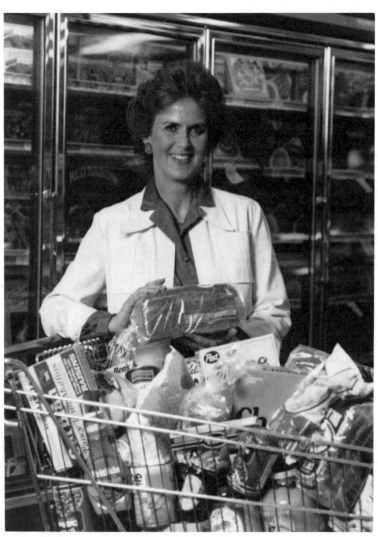

Jayne Benkendorf

ABOUT YOUR AUTHOR . . .
JAYNE BENKENDORF

CURRENT ACTIVITIES:

.Owner

PRODUCT RESEARCH SERVICE (PRS)
PRS does all the food research, evaluates food ingredients and researches grocery products for ingredients used. This research is the basis for which ratings are determined in *The Food Bible*.

Editor & Publisher

PRODUCT RESEARCH UPDATE
This is a monthly publication used to keep clients up to date on what is happening in the grocery store — including new foods coming on the market (the best foods and those to avoid) as well as food preparation and meal planning ideas direct from Jayne's kitchen. This service is designed for use in conjunction with *The Food Bible*.

Author

The Food Bible
The product of over four years research, including two years of actual field testing.

Lecturer

IN SEARCH OF THE GOOD FOODS
Jayne is a frequent lecturer and has conducted some 200 lectures over the past two years including: hospital and prenatal care groups, physicians' groups, medical research groups, and a guest speaker at universities, and she has appeared on radio and television talk shows.

Creator & Author	JAYNE'S QUICK & EASY RECIPES Sometimes referred to as the "Fabulous 30", these 30 recipes and meal plans feature high nutrient-dense meals, low in fat, sodium and cholesterol that take 15 minutes or less to get to the table.

PAST ACTIVITIES:

Counseling	Weight control and weight-control meal planning.
Teaching	Cooking and meal planning.
Registered Medical Technologist	Phlebotomist and Clinical Technician
Research	Oklahoma State University School of Veterinary Medicine.

THE FOOD BIBLE COMPANION

The very best combination for the informed grocery buyer - *The Food Bible* and **The Food Bible Companion.**

The Companion:

* Identifies new foods coming on the market - the best foods to buy and the foods to avoid.

* Advises on food preparation & meal planning direct from Jayne's kitchen.

* Provides quick & easy recipes - 15 minutes to the table.

* Highlights the very best foods offered in our grocery stores.

* Updates Jayne Benkendorf's latest research.

* And includes a special Feature Series each month.

For a complimentary issue, send **$1.00** (to cover postage & handling) to:

Jayne Benkendorf
P. O. Box 1828
Edmond, OK 73083-1828

THE FOOD BIBLE

For additional copies of *The Food Bible*, telephone TOLL FREE 1-800-356-9315. MasterCard/VISA accepted.

To order *The Food Bible* direct from the publisher, send your check or money order for $16.95 plus $2.75 shipping and handling ($19.70 postpaid) to Rainbow Books, Order Dept. 1-B, P.O. Box 1069, Moore Haven, Florida 33471-1069.

For QUANTITY PURCHASES, telephone Rainbow Books, 1-813-946-0293 or write to Rainbow Books, P.O. Box 1069, Moore Haven, Florida 33471-1069.